Carcinoma of the Esophagus

Contemporary Issues in Cancer Imaging

A Multidisciplinary Approach

Series Editors

Rodney H. Reznek

Cancer Imaging, St. Bartholomew's Hospital, London

Janet E. Husband

Diagnostic Radiology, Royal Marsden Hospital, Surrey

Current titles in the series

Cancer of the Ovary
Lung Cancer
Colorectal Cancer
Carcinoma of the Kidney

Forthcoming titles in the series

Carcinoma of the Bladder
Prostate Cancer
Squamous Cell Cancer of the Neck
Pancreatic Cancer
Interventional Radiological Treatment of Liver Tumours

Carcinoma of the Esophagus

Edited by

Sheila C. Rankin

Series Editors

Rodney H. Reznek

Janet E. Husband

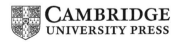

CAMBRIDGE
UNIVERSITY PRESS

CAMBRIDGE UNIVERSITY PRESS
Cambridge, New York, Melbourne, Madrid, Cape Town, Singapore, São Paulo

Cambridge University Press
The Edinburgh Building, Cambridge CB2 8RU, UK

Published in the United States of America by Cambridge University Press, New York

www.cambridge.org
Information on this title: www.cambridge.org/9780521882859

First published 2008

Printed in the United Kingdom at the University Press, Cambridge

A catalog record for this publication is available from the British Library

Library of Congress Cataloguing in Publication data
Carcinoma of the esophagus / edited by Sheila C. Rankin.
    p.   ;   cm. – (Contemporary issues in cancer imaging)
Includes bibliographical references and index.
ISBN 978-0-521-88285-9 (hardback : alk.paper)
1. Esophagus–Cancer.   2. Esophagus–Cancer–Diagnosis.   3. Esophagus–Cancer–Imaging.   I. Rankin,
Sheila, 1948-   II. Title.   III. Series.
[DNLM: 1. Esophageal Neoplasms–diagnosis.   2. Adenocarcinoma.   3. Carcinoma, Squamous Cell.
4. Diagnostic Imaging–methods.   5. Esophageal Neoplasms–theraphy.
WI 250 C2643 2008]
RC280.E8C367   2008
616.99′432–dc22   2007026633

ISBN 978-0-521-88285-9 hardback

Contents

Contributors

Andreas Adam, MB, BS (HONS), FRCP, FRCS,
FRCR, FFRRCSI (HON.)
Professor Interventional Radiology
Guy's, King's and St. Thomas' School
of Medicine
London, UK

Naama R. Bogot
Attending Radiologist
Department of Radiology
Hadassah Hebrew University Medical Center
Jerusalem, Israel

Lecturer
Department of Radiology
Division of Cardiothoracic Imaging
University of Michigan Health System, USA

Harriet M. R. Deere, MBBS, MRCPATH
Consultant Histopathologist
Department of Histopathology
Guy's and St. Thomas' Foundation Trust
London, UK

Peter Harper, FRCP
Consultant Medical Oncologist
Guy's and St. Thomas' Foundation Trust
London, UK

Jin-Yong Kang, MD, PHD, FRCP, FRCPED,
FRACP
Consultant Gastroenterologist and Honorary
Senior Lecturer
St. George's Hospital, London

David Landau, MRCP, FRCR
Consultant Clinical Oncologist
Guy's and St. Thomas' Foundation Trust
London, UK

Anne Marie Lennon, PHD, MRCP
Specialist Registrar
Lothian University Hospitals Division
Western General Hospital, Edinburgh

Laurence B. Lovat, BSC, PHD, FRCP
Consultant Gastroenterologist and Senior
Lecturer in Laser Medicine
National Medical Laser Centre
University College London Hospitals NHS
Foundation Trust
London, UK

Robert Mason, BSC, CHM, MD, FRCS
Consultant Upper GI Surgeon
Guy's and St. Thomas' Foundation Trust
St. Thomas' Hospital
London, UK

Satvinder S. Mudan, BSC, MD, FRCS
Consultant in Surgical Oncology
Royal Marsden Hospital
London, UK

Ian D. Penman, MD, FRCP EDIN
Consultant Gastroenterologist
Lothian University Hospitals Division
Western General Hospital, Edinburgh

Leslie Eisenbud Quint, MD
Professor of Radiology
Division of Cardiothoracic Imaging
University of Michigan Health System
Ann Arbor, Michigan, USA

Sheila C. Rankin, FRCR
Consultant Radiologist
Guy's and St. Thomas' Foundation Trust
London, UK

Tarun Sabharwal, FRCR, FRCSI
Consultant Interventional Radiologist and
Honorary Senior Lecturer
Guy's and St. Thomas' Foundation Trust
Department of Radiology
St. Thomas' Hospital
London, UK

Series foreword

Imaging has become pivotal in all aspects of the management of patients with cancer. At the same time, it is acknowledged that optimal patient care is best achieved by a multidisciplinary team approach. The explosion of technological developments in imaging over the past years has meant that all members of the multidisciplinary team should understand the potential applications, limitations, and advantages of all the evolving and exciting imaging techniques. Equally, to understand the significance of the imaging findings and to contribute actively to management decisions and to the development of new clinical applications for imaging, it is critical that the radiologist should have sufficient background knowledge of different tumors. Thus the radiologist should understand the pathology, the clinical background, the therapeutic options, and prognostic indicators of malignancy.

Contemporary Issues in Cancer Imaging: A Multidisciplinary Approach aims to meet the growing requirement for radiologists to have detailed knowledge of the individual tumors in which they are involved in making management decisions. A series of single subject issues, each of which will be dedicated to a single tumor site, edited by recognized expert guest editors, will include contributions from basic scientists, pathologists, surgeons, oncologists, radiologists, and others.

While the series is written predominantly for the radiologist, it is hoped that individual issues will contain sufficient varied information so as to be of interest to all medical disciplines and to other health professionals managing patients with cancer. As with imaging, advances have occurred in all these disciplines related to cancer management and it is our fervent hope that this series, bringing together expertise from such a range of related specialties, will not only promote the understanding and rational application of modern imaging but will also help to achieve the ultimate goal of improving outcomes of patient with cancer.

Rodney H. Reznek
London

Janet E. Husband
London

Preface to Carcinoma of the Esophagus

Esophageal cancer is a relatively uncommon but highly lethal malignancy. The incidence of adenocarcinoma is rapidly increasing, and improved survival will depend on prevention, earlier diagnosis, improved staging, and appropriate treatment.

As is the case with other malignancies, it is the multidisciplinary team approach toward patient care that determines the appropriate management of patients with esophageal cancer. For this approach to be effective, it is essential for all members of the multidisciplinary team to understand the role of imaging in esophageal cancer, its advantages, and limitations. Equally, it is vital for the radiologist to appreciate the clinical context of the imaging.

This volume provides a detailed review of new endoscopic methods of diagnosis, staging using both conventional and functional imaging, and assessment of surgical and medical methods of therapy.

Sheila C. Rankin

1

Epidemiology and Clinical Presentation in Esophageal Cancer

Satvinder S. Mudan and Jin-Yong Kang

Introduction

The esophagus begins at the level of the cricopharyngeus and traverses the length of the neck to pass through the mediastinum. It then pierces the right crus of the diaphragm and after a short abdominal component joins the stomach at the cardia. For descriptive purposes the esophagus is referred to as cervical (~6 cm), thoracic (~25 cm), and abdominal (~4 cm). Surgeons often refer to the esophagus in divisions of one-third, upper, middle, and distal, as this better relates to the operative options in esophagectomy.

Although not as common as cancer of other sites such as prostate, breast, and colorectum, esophageal cancer has a high lethality rate, the incidence being close to the cancer-specific mortality. Thus, in the USA in 2006, esophageal carcinoma was the 15th commonest cancer, with an estimated 14 550 cases, but it had the 8th highest mortality rate, with an estimated 13 770 deaths [1].

Esophageal cancer is remarkable for its marked variation by geographical region, ethnicity, and gender. There is a greater than tenfold difference in incidence rates between countries with a low incidence, for example, the United States, and those with a high incidence such as high-risk areas in Iran and China [2]. More than 90% of esophageal cancers are either squamous cell carcinomas (SCCs) or adenocarcinomas, with other tumor types such as melanomas, stromal tumors, lymphomas, or neuroendocrine cancers occurring only rarely in the esophagus. Most esophageal cancers occur in the lower and middle thirds, the cervical esophagus being an uncommon site of disease.

Although the presentation of SCC and adenocarcinoma of the esophagus in the patient are similar, the epidemiology, etiologoy, tumor biology, treatment strategies, and outcomes are quite different, and they are really two different diseases that occur in the same organ [3,4] (Table 1.1).

Carcinoma of the Esophagus, ed. Sheila C. Rankin. Published by Cambridge University Press. © Cambridge University Press 2008.

Table 1.1 Squamous cell carcinoma and adenocarcinoma of the esophagus: epidemiology, etiology, and symptoms

	Squamous cell carcinoma	Adenocarcinoma
Age	60–70 years, median 62.6 years	50–60 years, median 53.4 years
Sex	Male dominant, lower socioeconomic group	Male dominant, middle or upper socioeconomic group, 52% are university graduates
Associations	Head and neck cancer, smoking, alcohol excess and liver dysfunction, radiation exposure, achalasia, poor nutritional status, human papillomavirus (HPV) infection, *Helicobacter pylori* infection, Plummer–Vinson syndrome, tylosis palmaris, lye ingestion	Barrett's esophagus, gastroesophageal reflux disease, hiatus hernia, obesity, scleroderma, family history
Location	Mostly midesophagus (75% at level of tracheal bifurcation) and with a prominently linear growth pattern and wider nodal spread	Almost always distal one-third of esophagus (94% entirely subcarinal) and radial growth pattern with early local nodal dissemination
Symptoms and wider nodal spread	Progressive dysphagia, odynophagia, halitosis, unintentional weight loss, chest pain	Progressive dysphagia, odynophagia, halitosis, unintentional weight loss, chest pain

Epidemiology

The epidemiology of esophageal cancer in the Western world has changed dramatically over the last two decades. Up until the 1970s most esophageal cancers were of the squamous cell type, affecting mostly elderly men drawn from the poorer social classes and influenced by smoking and alcohol consumption. Since then there has been a dramatic increase in the incidence of adenocarcinoma, which tends to affect more affluent white men, often in their most productive years of life [2].

Squamous cell carcinoma

SCC of the esophagus remains in the top ten of cancers globally and represents a major healthcare problem. The marked geographical variation in incidence suggests that environmental factors are paramount in its causation. High-incidence regions of the world such as Southern and Eastern Africa, and a central Asian belt passing from Turkey through countries such as Iraq, Iran, and Kazakhstan and on to Northern China, are marked out by poverty and other poverty-related illnesses. The incidence in high-risk provinces can reach up to 100/10 000 per year compared to 5–10/10 000 per year in Western countries [2]. In the USA, SCC is more common among black people than among white people, but incidence rates have fallen by half across both groups between 1970 and 2000, with incidence rates of approximately 2/100 000 for white males and 10/100 000 for black people in 2000 [1,2,5]. These figures are probably related to increasing levels of wealth and education and reduction in exposure to causative agents.

The male : female ratio is 3:1 except in high-incidence areas where the distribution is more equal and reflects an equal exposure to risk factors [6]. Regional, socioeconomic, and racial variation within a country is demonstrated by a higher incidence of SCC in low income and low socioeconomic groups [5,7,8].

Adenocarcinoma

The last 30 years have seen a dramatic fall in the incidence of noncardia gastric cancer and, as mentioned earlier, a decline or stabilization in the incidence of SCC of the esophagus in Western countries [9,10,11,12,13]. Over the same period the age-standardized incidence of adenocarcinoma of the lower esophagus, previously a rare disease with incidence <1/100 000, has risen more rapidly than any other malignancy in the Western world. Since the mid 1990s its incidence has exceeded that for SCC [14,15,16]. The rise in incidence is most marked in the white male population, reaching about 5/100 000 for the white males in North America and 8–12/100 000 for white males in the highest incidence countries of Australia and the UK [7,13,17,18,19,20,21,22]. This represents an increase of about 400–800% from the 1970s and is about four times greater than the incidence for black males in the United States. The trend is similar for other North European countries [10,23,24,25]. Not only is the incidence higher in white males, but the annual increase in incidence, ~10% per year, is higher than for other racial groups and for white females, leading to an increasing sex and racial ratio [17,26,27]. The demographic distribution shows an age peak at 50–60 years and a male : female ratio between 2:1 and 12:1 [23]. Although it is possible that improved anatomic classification and histological verification might account for some of the time trends noted, the rapid changes point to a newly acquired etiological risk factor [10,13,14].

Etiology

Squamous cell carcinoma

Many of the environmental factors associated with a high incidence of SCC of the esophagus relate to poor socioeconomic circumstances. A diet rich in preserved and pickled foods and low in fresh fruit and vegetables, vitamin and mineral deficiencies, and a thermal effect of hot food and beverages have all been implicated. Alcohol intake and smoking are also strongly associated with an increased risk of SCC of the esophagus [28,29,30,31]. The risk is thought to be dose related and the genetic changes brought about by chronic exposure to causative agents lead to a progression through epithelial dysplasia and carcinoma *in situ* to invasive cancer [32]. After several years of cessation of exposure to irritant factors, such as smoking and alcohol, risk is substantially reduced [33]. Conditions such as caustic ingestion and achalasia of the cardia, which are associated with chronic mucosal inflammation, also predispose to SCC of the esophagus.

Adenocarcinoma

The recent and rapid escalation in incidence of esophageal adenocarcinoma would seem to suggest a mostly environmental rather than genetic effect. While a number of factors including race, obesity, use of esophageal sphincter-relaxing drugs, smoking, and alcohol consumption have all been incriminated as possible etiological factors in esophageal adenocarcinoma [34,35,36,37,38], many cohort studies have pointed strongly to gastroesophageal reflux and Barrett's disease (Barrett's esophagus) as a causative factor [39,40].

There is a strong dose–response relationship between previous gastroesophageal reflux symptoms and esophageal adenocarcinoma, but the relationship to cardia cancer is weaker [40]. Wu *et al.* demonstrated a threefold increase in esophageal cancer and a doubling in cardia cancer with reflux symptoms [41]. The relationship between adenocarcinoma of the lower esophagus and adenocarcinoma of the cardia is less clear. Siewert *et al.* have separated adenocarcinoma occurring at or near the gastroesophageal junction into three groups depending on the anatomic relation to the gastroesophageal junction. Type 1 tumors represent cancers of the lower esophagus, mostly arising in Barrett's esophagus. Type 2 and 3 tumors represent true cardia and proximal gastric cancers, respectively [42], and while their incidence has risen in recent decades, the changes are not as marked as for true lower esophageal adenocarcinoma that are associated with Barrett's esophagus, Type I. The clinical behavior and treatment of type 2 and 3 tumors are more like those of gastric carcinoma [43,44].

Gastroesophageal reflux leads to columnar cell metaplasia in the distal esophageal epithelium, a condition known as Barrett's esophagus. This increases the risk of developing esophageal adenocarcinoma 30- to 60-fold. The squamous cell epithelium of the normal esophagus is replaced with a mature columnar-type epithelium, with Barrett's mucosa being derived from pleuripotential cells in the basal layer of the esophageal epithelium [45,46,47]. The presence of goblet and pregoblet cells is a requisite for intestinal metaplasia, which is associated with the increased risk of malignant transformation. The probable driver toward metaplasia is that the columnar epithelium is more tolerant of refluxate and the progression to columnar metaplasia is a function of the refluxate content and periodicity [34]. Metaplasia of fundic- or cardiac-type gastric mucosa not involving the presence of goblet cells is thought to carry a lower risk of malignant transformation. Most cases of distal esophageal adenocarcinomas (90%) are thought to arise in the setting of Barrett's esophagus [48]. In other words, the risk of malignant transformation is greatly elevated in patients with Barrett's esophagus and much less elevated in patients with reflux esophagitis or nonerosive gastroesophageal reflux without Barrett's esophagus. Solaymani-Dodaran *et al.* reported relative risks for developing esophageal adenocarcinoma of 29.8 for Barrett's esophagus, 4.5 for reflux esophagitis, and 3.1 for gastroesophageal reflux without Barrett's esophagus or reflux esophagitis [39]. A patient with Barrett's esophagus has a 5% lifetime risk of developing esophageal adenocarcinoma. The risk of transformation from benign intestinal epithelium in Barrett's esophagus to dysplasia and then adenocarcinoma is related to the length of Barrett's epithelium lining the esophagus, duration of reflux disease, and presence of a hiatus hernia [49,50,51]. The risk of transformation may be mitigated by antireflux surgery, but the evidence is not strong enough to recommend this as a strategy for cancer prevention. Molecular markers of high risk are recognized but do not as yet form part of routine practice [52,53,54,55].

Dysplasia is classified as low or high grade and is characterized by the degree of hyperchromasia, nuclear:cytoplasm ratio, and glandular atypia. High-grade dysplasia is considered as indicative of at least an intraepithelial malignancy. About one-third of patients with high-grade dysplasia at biopsy will have invasive disease evident on a resection specimen. In population terms Barrett's esophagus is a common condition, occurring in 0.45–2.2% of all patients undergoing upper GI endoscopy, about 12% of patients undergoing endoscopy for reflux symptoms, and about 0.3% in unselected autopsy series [56]. While excess exposure to acid is demonstrable in most patients with Barrett's esophagus, progression to dysplasia is more likely in patients with alkaline or bile-containing duodenogastric reflux rather than those with pure acid reflux [57,58].

Several other potential causative factors have been evaluated. The incidence of esophageal adenocarcinoma has increased since the introduction of powerful acid suppressants such as histamine-2 receptor antagonists and proton pump inhibitors, but the lead time for carcinogenesis probably precludes these agents as etiological agents and the association is likely to reflect the use of these agents to treat symptoms of reflux in patients already at increased risk of developing esophageal adenocarcinoma. Drugs that reduce the lower esophageal sphincter tone, e.g., anticholingergics, nitroglycerin, beta-adrenergic agonists, aminophylline, and benzodiazepines, have all been implicated through increasing the potential for reflux [36]. Reduction in intragastric acidity through gastric mucosal atrophy-induced hypochlorhydria from *Helicobacter pylori* infection may be another factor in the promotion of distal esophageal SCC, while its carcinogenic effect in noncardia gastric cancer is well recognized. By contrast, *Helicobacter pylori* infection, especially of the cagA$^+$ strain, may have a protective effect against esophageal adenocarcinoma [59,60]. The role of diet is controversial, and while there appears to be an association with noncardia gastric cancer, the link to esophageal cancer is not so clear [61,62,63,64]. The relationship to smoking is less clear than that for SCC. Increased abdominal pressure brought about by central obesity, sedentary posture, and tight belts has also been implicated [37,65], although a high body mass index appears to be an independent risk factor for adenocarcinoma but not SCC [38].

Familial clustering has been demonstrated in Barrett's esophagus and adenocarcinoma of the esophagus, but no "Barrett gene" has been identified, and it is not clear whether the familial tendency represents a genetic predisposition or merely the effect of similar lifestyle factors among family members [66].

The carcinogenic pathway from Barrett's mucosa involves a multistep alteration in the genotype, loss of regulatory function, induction of proinflammatory enzymes such as cyclooxygenase-2, and angiogenesis. Consequently, chemoprevention and treatment through the use of therapies directed at specific molecular targets has been postulated [67].

Clinical presentation

The majority of symptomatic patients turn out to have advanced disease. Presenting symptoms are similar for SCC and adenocarcinoma. The most common are dysphagia and odynophagia (i.e., pain on swallowing). The pliability of the esophagus is such that dysphagia occurs when the lumen is obstructed by about 75% of the circumference, although a small tumor may cause a tight stenosis through intense fibrosis. Chronic cough secondary to laryngopharyngeal reflux may be an early marker of malignant transformation in Barrett's esophagus [68]. Hoarseness or Horner's syndrome usually implies invasion of the recurrent laryngeal nerve or cervical ganglia, and such patients are almost always inoperable. Cervical or supraclavicular lymphadenopathy is indicative of distant spread and indicates inoperability in adenocarcinoma. It is present in about one-third of SCCs, and resection with curative intent might still be considered in this disease with radical three-field node dissection, in particular for mid- or upper-third tumors [68].

Prognosis

While some rare esophageal tumors such as lipomas or smooth muscle tumors have a good outlook, the prognosis for SCC and adenocarcinoma of the esophagus is poor with an overall tumor-specific lethality rate of ~0.95 [69]. Survival appears comparable across age groups, but females appear to have better outcomes. For patients undergoing operations with curative intent, the 5-year survival ranges from 5 to 20%. Large tumors, nodal involvement, and extracapsular nodal spread are all strong prognostic factors for poor outcome [70]. Progression of nodal disease to subdiaphragmatic sites is generally considered to carry the same prognostic significance as distant metastases, although long-term survival with resection of celiac nodes is possible. It is likely that micrometastases in lymph nodes and sites such as bone marrow behave in a way different from clinically obvious disease.

Whether the type of operation performed affects outcome is uncertain. Tumor location in the upper esophagus predicates for a poor operative risk. Since most SCCs are either mid or upper esophageal cancers and other comorbidities such as age, chronic respiratory disease, liver disease, and poor nutrition are common, the immediate results of surgery are consistently worse for SCC than for adenocarcinoma [4,71,72]. Resections with microscopic positive surgical margins consistently perform worse than those with negative margins.

Cancer-specific outcomes have improved [73] in the last two decades through reduced surgical morbidity and mortality brought about by improvement in the perioperative care, multidisciplinary collaboration, and the use of multimodal therapies [74]. Although no survival advantage has been consistently demonstrated by adjuvant chemotherapy in resected esophageal cancer and trials of neoadjuvant chemotherapy or chemoradiotherapy are inconsistent, a large recently published British Medical Research Council study (ST-02 MAGIC study) demonstrated a significant tumor-specific survival advantage [75,76,77,78], and a distal esophageal location and a measurable response to preoperative chemotherapy appear to identify a favorable group [74,79,80,81]. Strategies based on identification of high-risk individuals allowing surveillance by endoscopy or molecular markers and for those progressing to cancer-targeted therapies with newer systemic agents and pretreatment response prediction are awaited [67,82,83,84,85].

Conclusions

The epidemiology of esophageal cancer is rapidly changing. In Western countries, adenocarcinoma of the lower esophagus has overtaken the previously more prevalent SCC. The divergent etiology and tumor behavior between the two diseases require different prevention and treatment strategies. Until its etiology becomes better understood, the continued rise in incidence of esophageal adenocarcinoma presents a significant healthcare problem in Western countries. Better identification of those at risk, e.g., individuals with Barrett's esophagus, might allow more effective screening policies. At present, surgery, when possible, represents the only potentially curative modality, but results remain poor and we await improvements in outcome through incorporation of therapies directed at novel cellular and molecular targets.

REFERENCES

1. A. Jemal, R. Siegel, E. Ward, *et al.* Cancer statistics, 2006. *CA Cancer J Clin*, **56** (2006), 106–30.
2. R. Holmes and T. L. Vaughan. Epidemiology and pathogenesis of esophageal cancer. *Semin Radiat Oncol*, **17** (2007), 2–9.
3. C. Mariette, L. Finzi, G. Piessen, *et al.* Esophageal carcinoma: prognostic differences between squamous cell carcinoma and adenocarcinoma. *World J Surg*, **29** (2005), 39–45.
4. J. R. Siewert and K. Ott. Are squamous and adenocarcinomas of the esophagus the same disease? *Semin Radiat Oncol*, **17** (2007), 38–44.
5. L. M. Brown, R. Hoover, D. Silverman, *et al.* Excess incidence of squamous cell esophageal cancer among US black men: role of social class and other risk factors. *Am J Epidemiol*, **153** (2001), 114–22.
6. H. R. Wabinga, D. M. Parkin, F. Wabwire-Mangen, and S. Nambooze. Trends in cancer incidence in Kyadondo County, Uganda, 1960–1997. *Br J Cancer*, **82** (2000), 1585–92.

7. A. Kubo and D. A. Corley. Marked regional variation in adenocarcinomas of the esophagus and the gastric cardia in the United States. *Cancer*, **95** (2002), 2096–102.

8. X. Wu, V. W. Chen, B. Ruiz, *et al*. Incidence of esophageal and gastric carcinomas among American Asians/Pacific Islanders, whites, and blacks: subsite and histology differences. *Cancer*, **106** (2006), 683–92.

9. S. Keeney and T. L. Bauer. Epidemiology of adenocarcinoma of the esophagogastric junction. *Surg Oncol Clin N Am*, **15** (2006), 687–96.

10. A. P. Vizcaino, V. Moreno, R. Lambert, *et al*. Time trends incidence of both major histologic types of esophageal carcinomas in selected countries, 1973–1995. *Int J Cancer*, **99** (2002), 860–8.

11. M. Pera. Trends in incidence and prevalence of specialized intestinal metaplasia, Barrett's esophagus, and adenocarcinoma of the gastroesophageal junction. *World J Surg*, **27** (2003), 999–1008.

12. M. Pera, C. Manterola, O. Vidal, and L. Grande. Epidemiology of esophageal adenocarcinoma. *J Surg Oncol*, **92** (2005), 151–9 (Review).

13. A. Newnham, M. J. Quinn, P. Babb, J. Y. Kang, and A. Majeed. Trends in the subsite and morphology of oesophageal and gastric cancer in England and Wales 1971–1998. *Aliment Pharmacol Ther*, **17** (2003), 665–76.

14. H. Pohl and H. G. Welch. The role of overdiagnosis and reclassification in the marked increase of esophageal adenocarcinoma incidence. *J Natl Cancer Inst*, **97** (2005), 142–6.

15. N. J. Shaheen. Advances in Barrett's esophagus and esophageal adenocarcinoma. *Gastroenterology*, **128** (2005), 1554–66 (Review).

16. J. Lagergren. Adenocarcinoma of oesophagus: what exactly is the size of the problem and who is at risk? *Gut*, **54**:Suppl. 1 (2005), 1–5 (Review).

17. A. Kubo and D. A. Corley. Marked multi-ethnic variation of esophageal and gastric cardia carcinomas within the United States. *Am J Gastroenterol*, **99** (2004), 582–8.

18. E. Bollschweiller, E. Wolfgarten, C. Gutschow, *et al*. Demographic variations in the rising incidence of esophageal adenocarcinoma in white males. *Cancer*, **92** (2001), 549–55.

19. R. V. Lord, M. G. Law, R. L. Ward, *et al*. Rising incidence of oesophageal adenocarcinoma in men in Australia. *J Gastroenterol Hepatol*, **13** (1998), 356–62.

20. A. Newnham, M. J. Quinn, P. Babb, J. Y. Kang, and A. Majeed. Trends in oesophageal and gastric cancer incidence, mortality and survival in England and Wales 1971–1998/1999. *Aliment Pharmacol Ther*, **17** (2003), 655–64.

21. S. S. Devesa, W. J. Blot, and J. F. Fraumeni. Changing patterns in the incidence of esophageal and gastric carcinoma in the United States. *Cancer*, **83** (1998), 2049–53.

22. Thames Cancer Registry. *Cancer in South East England 1997* (London: Thames Cancer Registry, 2000).

23. A. A. Botterweck, L. J. Schouten, A. Volovics, *et al*. Trends in incidence of adenocarcinoma of the oesophagus and gastric cardia in ten European countries. *Int J Epidemiol*, **29** (2000), 645–54.

24. B. P. Wijnhoven, M. W. Louwman, H. W. Tilanus, and J. W. Coebergh. Increased incidence of adenocarcinomas at the gastro-oesophageal junction in Dutch males since the 1990s. *Eur J Gastroenterol Hepatol*, **14** (2002), 115–22.

25. L. E. Hansson, P. Sparen, and O. Nyren. Increasing incidence of both major histological types of esophageal carcinomas among men in Sweden. *Int J Cancer*, **54** (1993), 402–7.

26. J. Powell, C. C. McConkey, E. W. Gillison, *et al*. Continuing rising trend in oesophageal adenocarcinoma. *Int J Cancer*, **102** (2002), 422–7.

27. M. Younes, D. E. Henson, A. Ertan, *et al*. Incidence and survival trends of esophageal carcinoma in the United States: racial and gender differences by histological type. *Scand J Gastroenterol*, **37** (2002), 1359–65.

28. L. S. Engel, W. H. Chow, T. L. Vaughan, *et al*. Population attributable risks of esophageal and gastric cancers. *J Natl Cancer Inst*, **95** (2003), 1404–13.

29. M. Farhadi, Z. Tahmasebi, S. Merat, *et al*. Human papillomavirus in squamous cell carcinoma of esophagus in a high-risk population. *World J Gastroenterol*, **11** (2005), 1200–3.

30. S. Bahmanyar and W. Ye. Dietary patterns and risk of squamous-cell carcinoma and adenocarcinoma of the esophagus and adenocarcinoma of the gastric cardia: a population-based case-control study in Sweden. *Nutr Cancer*, **54** (2006), 171–8.

31. H. Boeing, T. Dietrich, K. Hoffman, *et al*. Intake of fruits and vegetables and risk of cancer of the upper aero-digestive tract: the prospective EPIC-study. *Cancer Causes Control*, **17** (2006), 957–69.

32. H. Kuwano, H. Kato, T. Miyazaki, *et al*. Genetic alterations in esophageal cancer. *Surg Today*, **35** (2005), 7–18.

33. C. H. Lee, J. M. Lee, D. C. Wu, *et al*. Independent and combined effects of alcohol intake, tobacco smoking and betel quid chewing on the risk of esophageal cancer in Taiwan. *Int J Cancer*, **113** (2005), 456–63.

34. S. R. DeMeester and T. R. DeMeester. Columnar mucosa and intestinal metaplasia of the esophagus: fifty years of controversy. *Ann Surg*, **231** (2000), 303–21 (Review).

35. S. R. DeMeester. Adenocarcinoma of the esophagus and cardia: a review of the disease and its treatment. *Ann Surg Oncol*, **13** (2006), 12–30.

36. J. Lagergren, R. Bergstrom, H. O. Adami, and O. Nyren. Association between medications that relax the lower esophageal sphincter and risk for esophageal adenocarcinoma. *Ann Intern Med*, **133** (2000), 165–75.

37. J. Lagergren and C. Jansson. Use of tight belts and risk of esophageal adenocarcinoma. *Int J Cancer*, **119** (2006), 2464–6.

38. J. Lagergren, R. Bergstrom, and O. Nyren. Association between body mass and adenocarcinoma of the esophagus and gastric cardia. *Ann Intern Med*, **130** (1999), 883–90.

39. M. Solaymani-Dodaran, R. F. Logan, J. West, *et al*. Risk of oesophageal cancer in Barrett's oesophagus and gastro-oesophageal reflux. *Gut*, **53** (2004), 1070–4.

40. J. Lagergren, R. Bergstrom, A. Lindgren, and O. Nyren. Symptomatic gastroesophageal reflux as a risk factor for esophageal adenocarcinoma. *N Engl J Med*, **340** (1999), 825–31.

41. A. H. Wu, C. C. Tseng, and L. Bernstein. Hiatal hernia, reflux symptoms, body size, and risk of esophageal and gastric adenocarcinoma. *Cancer*, **98** (2003), 940–8.

42. J. R. Siewert and H. J. Stein. Classification of adenocarcinoma of the oesophagogastric junction. *Br J Surg*, **85** (1998), 1457–9.

43. J. R. Siewert, M. Feith, and H. J. Stein. Biologic and clinical variations of adenocarcinoma at the esophago-gastric junction: relevance of a topographic–anatomic subclassification. *J Surg Oncol*, **90** (2005), 139–46.

44. V. W. Rusch. Are cancers of the esophagus, gastroesophageal junction, and cardia one disease, two, or several? *Semin Oncol*, **31** (2004), 444–9.

45. H. M. Shields, S. J. Rosenberg, F. R. Zwas, *et al.* Prospective evaluation of multilayered epithelium in Barrett's esophagus. *Am J Gastroenterol*, **96** (2001), 3268–78.

46. J. Mueller, M. Werner, and M. Stolte. Barrett's esophagus: Histopathologic definitions and diagnostic criteria. *World J Surg*, **28** (2004), 148–54.

47. P. A. Atherford and J. A. Jankowski. Molecular biology of Barrett's cancer. *Best Pract Res Clin Gastroenterol*, **20** (2006), 813–27.

48. J. Theisen, H. J. Stein, H. Feith, *et al.* Preferred location for the development of esophageal adenocarcinoma within a segment of intestinal metaplasia. *Surg Endosc*, **20** (2006), 235–8.

49. N. J. Shaheen. Should we worry about the length of Barrett's esophagus? *Gastrointest Endosc*, **62** (2005), 682–5.

50. P. J. F. De Jonge, E. W. Steyerberg, E. J. Kuipers, *et al.* Risk factors for the development of esophageal adenocarcinoma in Barrett's esophagus. *Am J Gastroenterol*, **101** (2006), 1421–9.

51. B. Avidan, A. Sonnenberg, T. G. Schnell, *et al.* Hiatal hernia size, Barrett's length, and severity of acid reflux are all risk factors for esophageal adenocarcinoma. *Am J Gastroenterol*, **7** (2002), 1930–6.

52. D. V. Gopal, D. A. Lieberman, N. Margaret, *et al.* Risk factors for dysplasia in patients with Barrett's esophagus. *Dig Dis Sci*, **48** (2003), 1537–41.

53. A. P. Weston, P. Sharma, S. Mathur, *et al.* Risk stratification of Barrett's esophagus: Updated prospective multivariate analysis. *Am J Gastroenterol*, **99** (2004), 1657–66.

54. S. Oberg, J. Wenner, J. Johansson, *et al.* Barrett's esophagus. Risk factors for progression to dysplasia and adenocarcinoma. *Ann Surg*, **242** (2005), 49–54.

55. B. J. Ried, D. S. Levine, G. Longton, *et al.* Predictors of progression to cancer in Barrett's esophagus: Baseline histology and flow cytometry identify low and high risk patient subsets. *Am J Gastroenterol*, **95** (2000), 1669–76.

56. A. J. Cameron. Epidemiology of columnar lined esophagus and adenocarcinoma. *Gastroenterol Clin North Am*, **92** (1997), 918–22.

57. P. Singh, R. H. Taylor, and D. G. Colin-Jones. Esophageal motor dysfunction and acid exposure in reflux esophagitis are more severe if Barrett's metaplasia is present. *Am J Gastroenterol*, **89** (1994), 349–56.

58. D. S. Oh, J. A. Hagen, M. Fein, *et al.* The impact of reflux composition on mucosal injury and esophageal function. *J Gastrointest Surg*, **10** (2006), 787–96.

59. W. Ye, M. Held, J. Lagergren, *et al.* *Helicobacter pylori* infection and gastric atrophy: risk of adenocarcinoma and squamous-cell carcinoma of the esophagus and adenocarcinoma of the gastric cardia. *J Natl Cancer Inst*, **96** (2004), 388–96.

60. F. Kamanger, S. M. Dawsey, M. J. Blaser, *et al.* Opposing risks of gastric cardia and noncardia gastric adenocarcinomas associated with *Helicobacter pylori* seropositivity. *J Natl Cancer Inst*, **98** (2006), 1432–4.

61. C. A. González, P. Jakszyn, G. Pera, *et al.* Meat intake and risk of stomach and esophageal adenocarcinoma within the European Prospective Investigation into Cancer and Nutrition (EPIC). *J Natl Cancer Inst*, **98** (2006), 345–54.

62. C. A. González, G. Pera, A. Agudo, *et al.* Fruit and vegetable intake and the risk of stomach and oesophagus adenocarcinoma in the European Prospective Investigation into Cancer and Nutrition (EPIC-EURGAST). *Int J Cancer*, **118** (2006), 2559–66.

63. P. Jakszyn and C. A. Gonzalez. Nitrosamine and related food intake and gastric and oesophageal cancer risk: a systematic review of the epidemiological evidence. *World J Gastroenterol*, **12** (2006), 4296–303 (Review).

64. S. T. Mayne, H. A. Risch, R. Dubrow, *et al.* Nutrient intake and risk of subtypes of esophageal and gastric cancer. *Cancer Epidemiol Biomarkers Prev*, **10** (2001), 1055–62.

65. C. La Vecchia, E. Negri, P. Lagiou, and D. Trichopoulos. Oesophageal adenocarcinoma: a paradigm of mechanical carcinogenesis? *Int J Cancer*, **102** (2002), 269–70.

66. A. Chak, T. Lee, M. F. Kinnard, *et al.* Familial aggregation of Barrett's oesophagus, oesophageal adenocarcinoma, and oesophagogastric junctional adenocarcinoma in Caucasian adults. *Gut*, **51** (2002), 323–8.

67. W. P. Tew, D. P. Kelsen, and D. H. Ilson. Targeted therapies for esophageal cancer. *Oncologist*, **10** (2005), 590–601.

68. K. M. Reavis, C. D. Morris, D. V. Gopal, *et al.* Laryngopharyngeal reflux symptoms better predict the presence of esophageal adenocarcinoma than typical gastroesophageal reflux symptoms. *Ann Surg*, **239** (2004), 849–58.

69. S. M. Lagarde, F. J. W. ten Kate, J. B. Reitsma, *et al.* Prognostic factors in adenocarcinoma of the esophagus or gastroesophageal junction. *J Clin Oncol*, **24** (2006), 4347–55.

70. T. Lerut, W. Coosemans, G. Decker, *et al.* Extracapsular lymph node involvement is a negative prognostic factor in T3 adenocarcinoma of the distal esophagus and gastroesophageal junction. *J Thorac Cardiovasc Surg*, **126** (2003), 1121–8.

71. A. Alexandrou, P. A. Davis, S. Law, *et al.* Squamous cell carcinoma and adenocarcinoma of the lower third of the esophagus and gastric cardia: similarities and differences. *Dis Esophagus*, **15** (2002), 290–5.

72. H. Abunasra, S. Lewis, L. Beggs, *et al.* Predictors of operative death after oesophagectomy for carcinoma. *Br J Surg*, **92** (2005), 1029–33.

73. T. Lerut, W. Coosemans, G. Decker, *et al.* Diagnosis and therapy in advanced cancer of the esophagus and the gastroesophageal junction. *Curr Opin Gastroenterol*, **22** (2006), 437–41.

74. M. Koshy, N. Esiashvilli, J. C. Landry, *et al.* Multiple management modalities in esophageal cancer: combined modality management approaches. *Oncologist*, **9** (2004), 147–59.

75. M. Stahl. Adjuvant chemoradiotherapy in gastric cancer and carcinoma of the oesophago-gastric junction. *Onkologie*, **27** (2004), 33–6.

76. R. A. Malthaner, R. K. Wong, R. B. Rumble, *et al.* Neoadjuvant or adjuvant therapy for resectable esophageal cancer: a systematic review and meta-analysis. *BMC Med*, **2**:1 (2004), 35.

77. S. E. Greer, P. P. Goodney, J. E. Sutton, and J. D. Birkmeyer. Neoadjuvant chemoradiotherapy for esophageal carcinoma: a meta-analysis. *Surgery*, **137** (2005), 172–7.

78. D. Cunningham, W. H. Allum, S. P. Stenning, *et al.* Perioperative chemotherapy versus surgery alone for gastroesophageal cancer. *N Engl J Med*, **355** (2006), 11–20.

79. M. Stahl, H. Wilke, M. Stuschke, *et al.* Clinical response to induction chemotherapy predicts local control and long-term survival in multimodal treatment of patients with locally advanced esophageal cancer. *J Cancer Res Clin Oncol*, **131** (2005), 67–72.

80. R. J. Korst, A. L. Kansler, J. L. Port, *et al.* Downstaging of T or N predicts long-term survival after preoperative chemotherapy and radical resection for esophageal carcinoma. *Ann Thorac Surg*, **82** (2006), 480–4.

81. R. A. Malthaner, S. Collins, and D. Fenlon. Preoperative chemotherapy for resectable thoracic esophageal cancer. *Cochrane Database Syst Rev*, **3** (2006), CD001556.

82. E. S. Dellon and N. J. Shaheen. Does screening for Barrett's esophagus and adenocarcinoma of the esophagus prolong survival? *J Clin Oncol*, **23** (2005), 4478–82.

83. J. Tabernero, T. Macarulla, F. J. Ramos, and J. Baselga. Novel targeted therapies in the treatment of gastric and esophageal cancer. *Ann Oncol*, **16** (2005), 1740–8.

84. M. Akilu and D. H. Ilson. Targeted agents and esophageal cancer – the next step? *Semin Radiat Oncol*, **17** (2007), 62–9.

85. R. Langer, K. Specht, K. Becker, *et al.* Association of pretherapeutic expression of chemotherapy-related genes with response to neoadjuvant chemotherapy in Barrett carcinoma. *Clin Cancer Res*, **11** (2005), 7462–9.

2

Pathology of Esophageal Cancer

Harriet M. R. Deere

Introduction

Worldwide, squamous cell carcinoma is the most common malignant epithelial tumor of the esophagus. The majority of remaining tumors are adenocarcinomas, the incidence of which has been increasing dramatically in the last few decades in the Western world. Rarely, adenosquamous carcinoma and small cell carcinoma may occur.

This chapter will focus on the morphologic features of esophageal carcinoma and associated precursor lesions.

Histopathology of tumor types

Squamous cell carcinoma

Precursor lesions – hyperplasia and dysplasia

Squamous cell carcinoma is thought to develop through a multistep process from basal hyperplasia due to chronic esophagitis through increasing severity of dysplasia to invasion [1].

Dysplasia is defined as the presence of unequivocal neoplastic cells confined to the epithelium. It is seen more commonly in high cancer risk areas, e.g., China [2], is frequently seen adjacent to invasive carcinomas, and is often multifocal [3].

Traditionally, dysplasia has been classified as mild, moderate, or severe (and carcinoma *in situ*). More recently, a two-grade system for dysplasia in the gastrointestinal tract is preferred, with mild and moderate atypia being classed as low grade and severe dysplasia and carcinoma *in situ* as high grade.

The risk of carcinoma rises with increasing severity of dysplasia. A recent study from China has shown a relative risk of 2.9 for mild dysplasia, 9.8 for moderate, 28.3 for severe, and 34.4 for carcinoma *in situ* at 13 years follow-up [4].

Carcinoma of the Esophagus, ed. Sheila C. Rankin. Published by Cambridge University Press. © Cambridge University Press 2008.

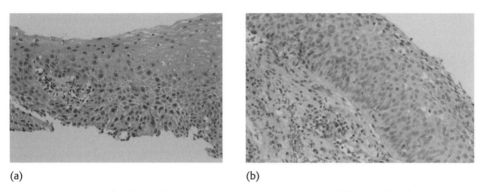

(a)   (b)

Figure 2.1 Squamous dysplasia of the esophagus: (a) mild dysplasia and (b) severe dysplasia.

Macroscopic appearance

At endoscopy, dysplastic epithelium may have an erythematous, friable appearance or be associated with erosions, nodules, or plaques [5]; however, it may appear normal.

Microscopic appearance

Dysplastic squamous epithelium shows cytological and architectural atypia, which varies in severity according to the grade. Architectural atypia refers to disorganization and loss of polarity of the cells and lack of surface maturation. Cytologically, the cells exhibit nuclear hyperchromasia (dark staining due to increased DNA), increased nuclear/cytoplasmic ratio, pleomorphism, and increased mitotic activity (Figure 2.1a and b).

Invasive squamous cell carcinoma

About 50–60% of squamous cell carcinomas occur in the middle third of the esophagus, approximately 30% occur in the lower third, and 10–20% in the upper third [6]. Squamous cell carcinomas are separated into superficial (early) and advanced tumors. Superficial tumors do not infiltrate beyond submucosa and may or may not have lymph node metastases. The incidence of superficial carcinoma is increasing, particularly in high-risk areas with screening programs. It accounts for 10–20% of tumors in Japan and less than 1% in Europe [7].

Macroscopic appearance

Superficial tumors may be plaque-like, polypoid, depressed, or occult [8]. Advanced tumors are exophytic (60%), ulcerating (25%), or infiltrative (15%). A

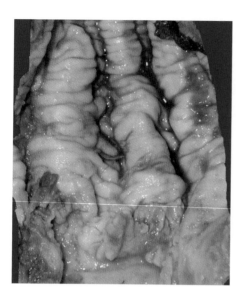

Figure 2.2 Infiltrative ulcerated squamous cell carcinoma. Case provided by Dr. F. Chang, London, United Kingdom.

combination of these patterns may be seen. Intramural metastases due to intramural lymphatic spread are found in 11–16% of cases [9,10], and multiple primary tumors are found in 14–31% of patients [11,12] (Figure 2.2).

Microscopic appearance

Squamous cell carcinoma is graded as well, moderately or poorly differentiated. Well-differentiated tumors show well-formed cell nests, squamous pearls with keratinization, and intercellular bridges. As tumors become less well differentiated the proportion of basaloid cells increases, there is increased nuclear pleomorphism and mitotic activity and loss of keratinization and prickle cells (Figure 2.3a and b).

Approximately two thirds of tumors are moderately differentiated, but it is common for there to be a variation in the degree of differentiation within a tumor.

Approximately 20–30% of tumors show focal glandular differentiation [13,14]. Focal neuroendocrine (small cell) differentiation is also sometimes seen [15].

Rare variants

Basaloid squamous cell carcinoma is similar to the tumor that more often occurs in the upper aerodigestive tract. Tumors are usually advanced at presentation. Prognosis appears similar to typical squamous cell carcinoma [16].

Spindle cell carcinoma (carcinosarcoma) usually presents as a large polypoid mass in the middle or lower third. Typically the tumors are biphasic, with conventional

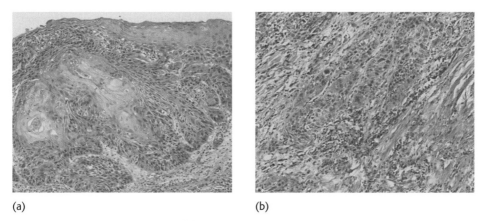

(a)   (b)

Figure 2.3 Squamous cell carcinoma: (a) well-differentiated squamous cell carcinoma and (b) poorly differentiated squamous cell carcinoma composed mainly of basaloid cells.

squamous cell carcinoma admixed with spindle cells showing variable differentiation. Presentation is often at an earlier stage due to the intraluminal growth. Prognosis is comparable to conventional squamous cell carcinoma of the same stage [17].

Verrucous squamous cell carcinoma presents as an exophytic papillary tumor. It is a very well-differentiated tumor that is notoriously difficult to diagnose on biopsy. Metastasis is rare; however; prognosis is poor as these tumors are locally aggressive and fistula formation may occur [18].

Differential diagnosis

It may sometimes be difficult to distinguish between reactive atypia due to inflammation and both dysplasia and invasive carcinoma, particularly on suboptimally orientated biopsy material. Chemoradiotherapy may also cause epithelial atypia. Reactive stromal cells in areas of ulceration may be worrying for malignancy, especially if there has been previous chemoradiotherapy. Cytokeratin staining is helpful in this situation as carcinoma is typically positive and mesenchymal cells are negative.

Adenocarcinoma

Precursor lesions – Barrett's esophagus and dysplasia

The most significant risk factor for adenocarcinoma is Barrett's esophagus.

Rarely, esophageal adenocarcinoma may arise from heterotopic gastric tissue [19,20] or the submucosal glands [21] and has a similar morphology to the Barrett's associated tumors.

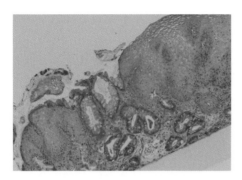

Figure 2.4 Columnar-lined esophagus. Columnar-lined esophagus with residual islands of squamous epithelium and intestinal metaplasia.

Barrett's esophagus refers to replacement of the normal esophageal squamous epithelium by metaplastic columnar epithelium as an acquired response to chronic acid and bile reflux. Three main types of columnar mucosa may be present and frequently coexist. The epithelium may be of junctional/cardiac type, gastric fundic type, or intestinal type with goblet cells (Figure 2.4).

It is the intestinal metaplastic epithelium that is a significant risk factor for malignancy.

The American College of Gastroenterology's definition of Barrett's esophagus is "a change in the esophageal epithelium of any length that can be recognized at endoscopy and is confirmed to have intestinal metaplasia by biopsy" [22]. In the United Kingdom, expert pathological opinion is that the identification of intestinal metaplasia should not be required for diagnosis and that the eponym Barrett's esophagus should be replaced by the term columnar-lined esophagus (CLE) [23]. The British view is that the absence of intestinal metaplasia on biopsy may be due to sampling error, as it has been shown that its demonstration is related to the number of biopsies taken [24].

Histological diagnosis of CLE requires close correlation with the endoscopic findings, as the microscopic features are not always pathognomonic. Biopsies are diagnostic for CLE when native esophageal structures, e.g., esophageal gland ducts are present, but these are only seen in approximately 15% of biopsies [25]. In their absence the pathologist can only corroborate the endoscopic diagnosis if columnar mucosa is present. Biopsy from the gastroesophageal junction or from a hiatus hernia, with or without intestinal metaplasia, may have a similar appearance. It is also important to distinguish between CLE and microscopic intestinal metaplasia at the cardia.

There have been conflicting results from studies looking at cytokeratin (CK7/20) staining patterns that may help distinguish CLE from intestinal metaplasia at the gastroesophageal junction/stomach [26,27,28].

The metaplastic epithelium is thought to originate from multipotential stem cells. The precise location of these cells is unclear; however, the gland ducts and basal epithelial layer are likely [29,30]. A distinctive multilayered epithelium with features of both squamous and columnar epithelium has been described and may represent a transitional phase in the conversion of squamous epithelium to CLE [31].

Approximately 5% of patients with CLE develop dysplasia, which is classified as low or high grade. An "indefinite for dysplasia" category is used for cases where it is not possible to distinguish between true dysplasia and reactive atypia due to inflammation.

Adenocarcinoma is found in 30–50% of resection specimens from patients with a biopsy diagnosis of high-grade dysplasia [32,33,34]. It is recommended that two pathologists confirm the diagnosis of high-grade dysplasia prior to treatment, one of whom should ideally be an expert gastrointestinal pathologist. Low-grade dysplasia may persist, regress to nonneoplastic metaplasia, or progress to high-grade dysplasia or carcinoma. High-grade dysplasia may also regress to low-grade dysplasia, but the majority of cases progress to carcinoma within 4 years [35,36].

Recent research has led to a greater understanding of the molecular alterations involved in neoplastic progression. Proliferation markers, aneuploidy, p53, p16, and adenomatous polyposis coli (APC) mutations, and cyclin D1 overexpression are some of the most common abnormalities investigated. However, currently there are no molecular techniques that are sufficiently reliable for routine use either for the diagnosis of dysplasia or to predict progression [23].

Macroscopic appearance
Columnar epithelium has a velvety red appearance. Often dysplastic epithelium appears endoscopically normal, but granularity, plaques, or erosions are sometimes present [37] (Figure 2.5).

Microscopic appearance
Dysplastic epithelium displays architectural abnormalities such as a villiform surface and crowding and budding of the glands. Cytological atypia includes nuclear hyperchromasia and pleomorphism, nuclear stratification, increased mitotic activity, and atypical mitoses. There is lack of surface maturation, with atypical cells extending onto the mucosal surface (Figure 2.6a and b).

Effects of treatment
Studies have shown that CLE may regress with antireflux surgery or medical treatment [38,39].

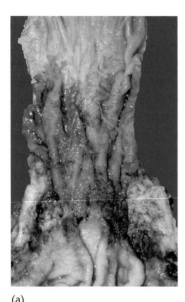

Figure 2.5 Distal esophageal adenocarcinoma arising on a background of columnar-lined esophagus. Case provided by Dr. F. Chang, London, United Kingdom.

(a)

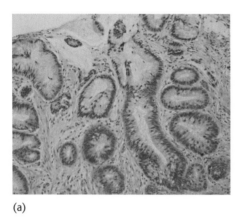

(a)

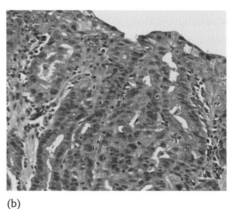

(b)

Figure 2.6 Columnar-lined esophagus. (a) Low-grade dysplasia. The nuclei are elongated, pseudostratified, and hyperchromatic. There is no surface maturation. (b) High-grade dysplasia. The glands are closely packed together and show cytological atypia with round nuclei with prominent nucleoli.

Endoscopic ablation techniques are increasingly used and also lead to squamous reepithelialization. This occurs due to extension of adjacent squamous epithelium and the formation of squamous islands arising from the submucosal gland ducts. Squamous metaplasia is often seen within metaplastic glands unrelated to esophageal ducts, lending support for the existence of multipotential stem cells [40].

Metaplastic or dysplastic glandular epithelium may persist beneath the new squamous epithelium; hence, deep biopsies are required on follow-up. Currently, the long-term behavior of this concealed glandular epithelium is unknown.

Invasive adenocarcinoma

Macroscopic appearance
Most tumors are advanced at the time of presentation and are ulcerating infiltrative lesions (Figure 2.6). They are less frequently exophytic (10–15%) compared with squamous cell carcinomas [41]. Rarely, they appear papillary or show diffuse infiltration resembling gastric linitis plastica [42].

Microscopic appearance
Adenocarcinomas are graded as well, moderately or poorly differentiated, according to the proportion of tumor cells forming glands (Figure 2.7a and b). Tumors can be mucinous with prominent extracellular mucin pools. Signet ring cell carcinoma is rare [43]. Very rarely, CLE-associated adenocarcinoma may have foci of admixed choriocarcinoma [44,45].

Small cell carcinoma

This accounts for approximately 1% of primary esophageal carcinomas [46]. It has a similar appearance to the more common pulmonary tumor and is highly aggressive.

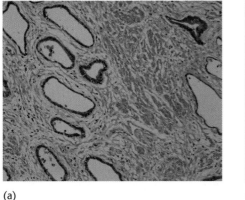
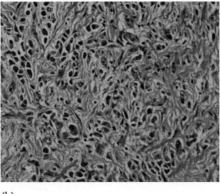

(a)   (b)

Figure 2.7 Invasive adenocarcinoma. (a) Well-differentiated adenocarcinoma composed of infiltrating glands with mild cytological atypia. (b) Poorly differentiated adenocarcinoma composed of sheets of cells without gland formation.

Staging

The TNM system is used for staging [47]. The Siewert classification is recommended for adenocarcinoma around the esophagogastric junction [48]. Tumors arising 1–5 cm above the junction (type 1) are staged with the esophageal TNM, whilst the gastric TNM system is recommended for tumors arising at the junction (type 2) or 2–5 cm below (type 3). Proformas have been developed to ensure that all relevant prognostic information is included in pathology reports [49,50].

Prognostic factors

Depth of tumor invasion is the most important and often the only independent prognostic indicator on multivariate analysis [41,51,52]. Lymph node metastasis is also a significant prognostic factor. The number of positive nodes and ratio of involved to uninvolved nodes have been found to be significant [53,54]. Vascular invasion and resection margin status have also been repeatedly shown to be significant on univariate analysis [41,51,55,56,57].

The histological type of tumor has not been shown to be significant in advanced disease, but several studies have shown a survival advantage for early (T1) adenocarcinoma compared to squamous cell carcinoma [58,59]. Other histological and molecular markers such as tumor grade, p53 and Her2 status, and ploidy do not appear to be independent predictors of poor prognosis [51,52,60,61].

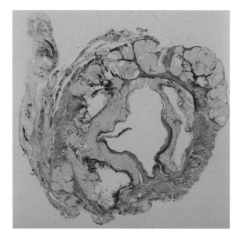

Figure 2.8 Effects of chemoradiotherapy. Acellular mucin pools throughout the esophageal wall in a treated adenocarcinoma.

Neoadjuvant treatment

As a consequence of the increasing use of preoperative chemoradiotherapy, resection specimens may often show the effects of this treatment. Systems for scoring the degree of regression exist but are rarely used in routine practice [62,63]. With response to therapy, ulceration, inflammation, fibrosis, and calcification are frequently seen. Sections may show only keratin surrounded by a foreign body giant cell reaction when a squamous cell carcinoma has regressed. Mucin pools are frequently seen in treated adenocarcinomas (Figure 2.8). Viable tumor may be present as small groups of cells, and these may show marked atypia due to the treatment. Cytokeratin staining is often required when only occasional tumor cells remain. Staging is based only on residual viable tumor. Tumor that has completely regressed would be staged as ypT0N0.

Conclusion

The role of the surgical pathologist has expanded from providing solely diagnostic information to include some important data regarding prognosis. At present this prognostic information is limited to histological factors with regard to esophageal tumors. Biological markers are been intensively studied in the research setting, and it is anticipated that these will be of increasing value in routine practice in determining prognosis and hopefully increase management options for these tumors.

REFERENCES

1. S. M. Dawsey, K. J. Lewin, G. Q. Wang, *et al.* Squamous esophageal histology and subsequent risk of squamous cell carcinoma of the esophagus. A prospective follow-up study from Linxian, China. *Cancer*, **74** (1994), 1686–92.

2. S. L. Qui and G. R. Yang. Precursor lesions of esophageal cancer in high-risk populations in Henan Province, China. *Cancer*, **62** (1998), 551–7.

3. M. Morita, H. Kuwano, M. Yasuda, *et al.* The multicentric occurrence of squamous epithelial dysplasia and squamous cell carcinoma in the oesophagus. *Cancer*, **74** (1994), 2889–95.

4. G. Q. Wang, C. C. Abnet, Q. Shen, *et al.* Histological precursors of oesophageal squamous cell carcinoma: results from a 13 year prospective follow up study in a high risk population. *Gut* **54** (2005), 187–92.

5. S. M. Dawsey, G. Q. Wang, W. M. Weinstein, *et al.* Squamous dysplasia and early esophageal cancer in the Linxian region of China: Distinctive endoscopic lesions. *Gastroenterology*, **105** (1993), 1333–40.

6. K. J. Lewin and H. D. Appelman. *Atlas of Tumor Pathology, 3rd Series, Fascicle 18. Tumors of the Esophagus and Stomach.* (Washington DC: Armed Forces Institute of Pathology, 1996).

7. P. Froelicher and G. Miller. The European experience with esophageal cancer limited to the mucosa and submucosa. *Gastrointest Endosc*, **32** (1986), 88–90.

8. W. V. Bogomoletz, G. Molas, B. Gayet, and F. Potet. Superficial squamous cell carcinoma of the esophagus. A report of 76 cases and review of the literature. *Am J Surg Pathol*, **13** (1989), 535–46.

9. H. Kato, Y. Tachimori, H. Watanabe, *et al.* Intramural metastasis of thoracic esophageal carcinoma. *Int J Cancer*, **50** (1992), 49–52.

10. H. Kuwano. Peculiar histopathologic features of esophageal cancer. *Surg Today*, **28** (1998), 573–5.

11. H. Kuwano, S. Ohno, H. Matsuda, *et al.* Serial histologic evaluation of multiple primary squamous cell carcinomas of the esophagus. *Cancer*, **61** (1988), 1635–8.

12. P. Pesko, S. Rakic, M. Milicevic, *et al.* Prevalence and clinicopathologic features of multiple squamous cell carcinoma of the esophagus. *Cancer*, **73** (1994), 2687–90.

13. H. Kuwano, H. Ueo, K. Sugimachi, *et al.* Glandular or mucus-secreting components in squamous cell carcinoma of the esophagus. *Cancer*, **56** (1985), 514–18.

14. K. Takubo, K. Sasajima, K. Yamashita, *et al.* Morphological heterogeneity of esophageal carcinoma. *Acta Pathol Jpn*, **39** (1989), 180–9.

15. Y. Fujiwara, K. Nakagawa, T. Tanaka, *et al.* Small cell carcinoma of the esophagus combined with superficial esophageal cancer. *Hepatogastroenterology*, **43** (1996), 1360–9.

16. M. Sarbia, P. Vereet, F. Bittinger, *et al.* Basaloid squamous carcinoma of the esophagus. Diagnosis and prognosis. *Cancer*, **79** (1997), 1871–8.

17. C. Du Boulay and P. Isaacson. Carcinoma of the oesophagus with spindle cell features. *Histopathology*, **5** (1981), 403–14.

18. P. Biemond, F. J. ten Kate, and M. van Blankenstein. Esophageal verrucous carcinoma: histologically a low-grade malignancy but a fatal disease. *J Clin Gastroenterol*, **13** (1991), 102–7.

19. W. N. Christensen and S. S. Sternberg. Adenocarcinoma of the upper esophagus arising in ectopic gastric mucosa; two case reports and review of the literature. *Am J Surg Pathol*, **11** (1987), 397–402.

20. G. Y. Lauwers, G. V. Scott, and G. N. Vauthey. Adenocarcinoma of the upper esophagus arising in cervical ectopic gastric mucosa: Rare evidence of malignant potential of so-called "inlet patch." *Dig Dis Sci*, **43** (1998), 901–7.

21. Y. Endoh, M. Miyawaki, G. Tamura, *et al.* Esophageal adenocarcinoma that probably originated in the esophageal gland duct: A case report. *Pathol Int*, **49** (1999), 156–9.

22. R. E. Sampliner. Practice guidelines on the diagnosis, surveillance and therapy of Barrett's esophagus. *Am J Gastroenterol*, **93** (1998), 1028–31.

23. A. Watson, R. C. Heading, and N. A. Shepherd. *Guidelines for Diagnosis and Management of Barrett's Columnar-Lined Oesophagus. A Report of the Working Party of the British Society of Gastroenterology.* (2005).

24. N. A. Shepherd and L. R. Biddlestone. The histopathology and cytopathology of Barrett's oeso-phagus. In *CPD Bulletin Cellular Pathology*, ed. S. Manek. (London: Rila Publications, 1999), **1**, 39–44.

25. K. Takubo, J. M. Nixon, and J. R. Jass. Ducts of esophageal glands proper and Paneth cells in Barrett's esophagus: frequency in biopsy specimens. *Pathology*, **27** (1995), 315–17.

26. I. A. Mohammed, C. J. Streutker, and R. H. Riddell. Utilization of cytokeratins 7 and 20 does not differentiate between Barrett's esophagus and gastric cardiac intestinal metaplasia. *Mod Pathol*, **15** (2002), 611–16.

27. R. D. Odze. Cytokeratin 7/20 immunostaining: Barrett's oesophagus or gastric intestinal meta-plasia. *Lancet*, **359** (2000), 1711–13.

28. A. H. Ormsby, J. R. Goldblum, and T. W. Rice, *et al.* Cytokeratin subsets can reliably distinguish Barrett's oesophagus from intestinal metaplasia of the stomach. *Hum Pathol*, **30** (1999), 288–94.

29. P. Gillen, P. Keeling, P. J. Byrne, *et al.* Experimental columnar metaplasia in the canine oeso-phagus. *Br J Surg*, **75** (1988), 113–15.

30. N. A. Wright. Migration of the ductular elements of gut-associated glands gives clues to the histogenesis of structures associated with responses to acid hypersecretory state: the origins of "gastric metaplasia" in the duodenum, of the specialized mucosa of Barrett's esophagus and of pseudopyloric metaplasia. *Yale J Biol Med*, **69** (1996), 147–53.

31. J. N. Glickman, Y. Y. Chen, H. H. Wang, *et al.* Phenotypic characteristics of a distinctive multi-layered epithelium suggests that it is a precursor in the development of Barrett's esophagus. *Am J Surg Pathol*, **25** (2001), 569–78.

32. N. K. Altorki, M. Sunagawa, A. G. Little, D. B. Skinner. High-grade dysplasia in the columnar lined esophagus. *Am J Surg*, **161** (1991), 97–9.

33. M. Pera, V. F. Trastek, H. A. Carpenter, *et al.* Barrett's esophagus with high-grade dysplasia: an indication for esophagectomy? *Ann Thorac Surg*, **54** (1992), 199–204.

34. E. E. Tseng, T. T. Wu, C. J. Yeo, and R. F. Heitmiller. Barrett's esophagus with high grade dysplasia: surgical results and long-term outcome – an update. *J Gastrointest Surg*, **7** (2003), 164–70.

35. M. Miros, P. Kerlin, and N. Walker. Only patients with dysplasia progress to adenocarcinoma in Barrett's oesophagus. *Gut*, **32** (1991), 1441–6.

36. P. Sharma, T. G. Morales, A. Bhattacharyya, *et al.* Relative risk of dysplasia for patients with intestinal metaplasia in the distal oesophagus and gastric cardia. *Gut*, **46** (1999), 9–13.

37. D. S. Levine. Management of dysplasia in the columnar-lined esophagus. *Gastroenterol Clin North Am*, **26** (1997), 613–34.

38. R. R. Gurski, J. H. Peters, J. A. Hagen, *et al.* Barrett's esophagus can and does regress after anti-reflux surgery: a study of prevalence and predictive features. *J Am Coll Surg*, **197** (2003), 882–3.

39. B. T. Cooper, W. Chapman, C. S. Neumann, and J. C. Gearty. Continuous treatment of Barrett's oesophagus patients with proton pump inhibitors up to 13 years: observations on regression and cancer incidence. *Aliment Pharmacol Ther*, **15** (2006), 727–33.

40. L. R. Biddlestone, C. P. Barham, S. P. Wilkinson, *et al.* The histopathology of treated Barrett's esophagus. Squamous re-epithelialization after acid suppression and laser and photo-dynamic therapy. *Am J Surg Pathol*, **22** (1998), 239–45.

41. F. Paraf, J. F. Flejou, J. P. Pignon, *et al.* Surgical pathology of adenocarcinoma arising in Barrett's esophagus. Analysis of 67 cases. *Am J Surg Pathol*, **19** (1995), 183–91.

42. G. Chejfec, V. R. Jablokow, and V. E. Gould. Linitis plastica carcinoma of the oesophagus. *Cancer*, **51** (1983), 2139–43.

43. M. Sarbia. The histological appearances of oesophageal adenocarcinoma – an analysis based on 215 resection specimens. *Virchows Arch*, **44** (2006), 532–8.

44. J. C. McKechnie and R. E. Fechner. Choriocarcinoma and adenocarcinoma of the esophagus with gonadotrophin secretion. *Cancer*, **27** (1971), 694–702.

45. S. H. Wasan, J. B. Schofiled, T. Krausz, *et al.* Combined choriocarcinoma and yolk sac tumour arising in Barrett's esophagus. *Cancer*, **73** (1994), 514–17.

46. F. Casas, F. Ferrer, B. Farrus, *et al.* Primary small cell carcinoma of the esophagus: A review of the literature with emphasis on therapy and prognosis. *Cancer*, **80** (1997), 1366–72.

47. F. L. Greene, D. L. Page, I. D. Fleming, *et al.*, eds. *AJCC Cancer Staging Manual*, 6th edn. (New York: Springer, 2002).

48. J. R. Siewert and H. J. Stein. Classification of adenocarcinoma of the oesophagogastric junction. *Br J Surg*, **85** (1998), 1457–9.

49. N. B. N. Ibrahim. ACP Best Practice No.155. Guidelines for handling oesophageal biopsies and resection specimens and their reporting. *J Clin Pathol*, **53** (2000), 89–94.

50. N. Mapstone. *Minimum Dataset for Oesophageal Carcinoma Histopathology Reports.* (London: The Royal College of Pathologists, 2006).

51. H. Ide, T. Nakamura, K. Hayashi, *et al.* Esophageal squamous cell carcinoma: pathology and prognosis. *World J Surg*, **18** (1994), 321–30.

52. S. S. Robey-Cafferty, A. K. el-Naggar, A. A. Sahin, *et al.* Prognostic factors in esophageal squamous carcinoma – a study of histologic features, blood-group expression, and DNA ploidy. *Am J Clin Pathol*, **95** (1991), 844–9.

53. Y. Gu, S. G. Swisher, J. A. Ajani, *et al.* The number of lymph nodes with metastasis predicts survival in patients with esophageal or esophagogastric junction adenocarcinoma who receive preoperative chemoradiation. *Cancer*, **106** (2006), 1017–25.

54. K. Kawahara, K. Maekawa, K. Okabayashi, *et al.* The number of lymph node metastases influences survival in esophageal cancer. *J Surg Oncol*, **67** (1998), 160–3.

55. S. P. Dexter, H. Sue-Ling, M. J. McMahon, *et al.* Circumferential resection margin involvement: an independent predictor of survival following surgery for oesophageal cancer. *Gut*, **48** (2001), 667–70.

56. P. M. Sagar, D. Johnston, M. J. McMahon, *et al.* Significance of circumferential resection margin involvement after oesophagectomy for cancer. *Br J Surg*, **80** (1993), 1386–8.

57. P. Theunissen, F. Borchard, and D. C. J. Poortvliet. Histopathological evaluation of oesophageal carcinoma. The significance of venous invasion. *Br J Surg*, **78** (1991), 930–2.

58. A. H. Holscher, E. Bollschweiler, P. M. Schneider, and J. R. Siewert. Prognosis of early esophageal cancer. Comparison between adeno-carcinoma and squamous-cell carcinoma. *Cancer*, **76** (1995), 178–86.

59. C. Mariette, L. Finzi, G. Piessen, *et al.* Esophageal carcinoma: prognostic differences between squamous cell carcinoma and adenocarcinoma. *World J Surg*, **29** (2005), 39–45.

60. A. Kanamoto, H. Kato, Y. Tachimori, *et al.* No prognostic significance of p53 expression in esophageal squamous cell carcinoma. *J Surg Oncol*, **72** (1999), 94–8.

61. Wang, K. C. Chow, K. H. Chi, *et al.* Prognosis of esophageal squamous cell carcinoma: Analysis of clinicopathological and biological factors. *Am J Gastroenterol*, **94** (1999), 1933–40.

62. S. J. Darnton, S. M. Allen, C. W. Edwards, and H. R. Matthews. Histopathological findings in oesophageal carcinoma with and without preoperative chemotherapy. *J Clin Pathol*, **46** (1993), 51–5.

63. A. M. Mandard, F. Dalibard, J. C. Mandard, *et al.* Pathologic assessment of tumour regression after preoperative chemo-radiotherapy of esophageal carcinoma. Clinicopathologic correlations. *Cancer*, **73** (1994), 2680–6.

3

Recent Advances in the Endoscopic Diagnosis of Esophageal Cancer

Anne Marie Lennon and Ian D. Penman

Introduction

Esophageal cancer is the seventh most common malignancy worldwide and has the sixth highest cancer mortality rate [1]. It has one of the most rapidly increasing incidence of all cancers in the last 5 years [2,3] and is associated with a poor 1 and 5-year survival in the UK [4].

Correct staging of esophageal cancer is essential for patient care. This not only gives a good indication of survival but also allows for optimum management of the patient. In patients with very early oesophageal cancer (Tis/T1m), local treatment with endoscopic mucosal resection (EMR) or photodynamic therapy can be considered. For those patients with more advanced disease (Stages IIB–III), many centers now advocate using neoadjuvant chemotherapy (OEO2) or chemoradiotherapy prior to surgery as this may improve survival [5,6]. For those patients with metastatic disease (Stage IV), palliative treatment is appropriate.

Endoscopic imaging

Flexible videoendoscopy with biopsy and/or brush cytology is the gold standard investigation for the diagnosis of esophageal carcinoma. Endoscopy is more sensitive and specific than double-contrast barium meal for the diagnosis of upper gastrointestinal cancer [7], and when biopsy and cytology are combined, the accuracy of endoscopy for diagnosis approaches 100% [8]. Rarely, in patients with pseudoachalasia and repeated negative mucosal biopsy, endoscopic ultrasound with or without fine-needle aspiration biopsy may provide supportive evidence for malignancy and a tissue diagnosis [9].

Carcinoma of the Esophagus, ed. Sheila C. Rankin. Published by Cambridge University Press. © Cambridge University Press 2008.

Table 3.1   Features to note at endoscopy on diagnosis of an esophageal cancer

1. Position relative to the incisor teeth (in centimeters) with proximal and distal margins
2. The morphology of the lesion using the Japanese–Bormann classification (Table 4) if the lesion is compatible with a superficial lesion
3. Presence and proximal extent of any Barrett's esophagus
4. Presence of a hiatal hernia
5. Involvement of the gastric cardia or extension along lesser curve
6. Presence of metastatic or synchronous lesions elsewhere in the upper gastrointestinal tract
7. Previous gastric or duodenal surgery

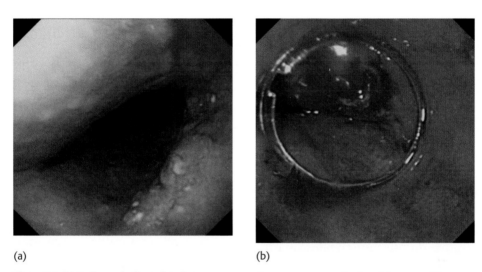

(a)   (b)

Figure 3.1 (a) Endoscopic view of early squamous carcinoma seen as a raised nodular area with superficial ulceration. (b) Early superficial (5 mm) adenocarcinoma arising in short-segment Barrett's esophagus just above the esophagogastric junction.

When a suspicious lesion is seen at endoscopy, it is important to document certain features (Table 3.1) that may provide important information for planning therapy and deciding between surgical resection, radiotherapy, and stent insertion. Lesions at the esophagogastric junction (EG junction) should be classified using the Siewert classification [10]: those which are predominantly in the esophagus are type 1 junctional; those that are mainly within the stomach are type 3; and those that are equally distributed between the esophagus and stomach as type 2.

Early esophageal cancer may appear as minor irregularities of the mucosa, areas of erythema, or depressed, raised, or ulcerated areas (Figure 3.1). Japanese

Table 3.2 Classification of superficial esophageal tumors using the Japanese system [12]

Type	Endoscopic appearance
Type 0	Superficial polypoid, flat/depressed, or excavated
Type 0-I	Polypoid
Type 0-Ip	Pedunculated
Type 0-Is	Sessile
Type 0-II	Nonpolypoid and nonexcavated
Type 0-IIa	Slightly elevated
Type 0-IIb	Completely flat
Type 0-IIc	Slightly depressed without ulcer
Type 0-III	Nonpolypoid with a frank ulcer
Type 1	Polypoid, usually attached to a wide base
Type 2	Ulcerated carcinomas with sharply demarcated and raised margins
Type 3	Ulcerated, infiltrating carcinomas without definite limits
Type 4	Nonulcerated, diffusely infiltrating carcinomas
Type 5	Unclassifiable advanced carcinomas

endoscopists have found that the endoscopic classification of a lesion can be an important determinant of whether endoscopic therapy, such as EMR, should be applied. They have attempted to identify this group of patients with minimally invasive disease, using endoscopic features [11]. Based on these features, the tumor can be divided into types 0 to 5, where type 0 corresponds with a minimally invasive tumor and type 4 with a diffusely infiltrating cancer (Table 3.2). Type 0 tumors are further subdivided based on their endoscopic appearance into types 0-I, 0-II, and 0-III, with types 0-I and 0-II further subdivided. A detailed description, with illustration of different endoscopic staging features, can be found elsewhere [12].

Dysplasia or early esophageal cancer can be difficult to detect even for an experienced endoscopist. This is because lesions are often subtle, presenting as small erosive or flat plaques. The use of four-quadrant biopsies in Barrett's esophagus has a low sensitivity, as high-grade intraepithelial neoplasia (HGIN) and early adenocarcinoma are often multifocal and flat. New techniques have therefore been developed, which highlight dysplastic or neoplastic lesions through a variety of methods.

Chromoendoscopy

Chromoendoscopy involves the use of agents that enhance the distinction between diseased and normal mucosa, either by filling surface crevices or by differential uptake by diseased epithelium. Many chromoendoscopy agents have been studied in the detection of esophageal carcinoma, of which Lugol's iodine and methylene blue have been most widely studied.

Lugol's iodine

Lugol's iodine contains iodine and potassium iodine and has an affinity for glycogen in nonkeratinized squamous epithelium. Normal squamous epithelium stains black or dark brown. This contrasts with inflamed, dysplastic, or malignant cells, which are glycogen depleted and consequently appear minimally stained or unstained (Figure 3.2) [13]. About 1–3% Lugol's iodine is sprayed onto the mucosa by using a standard washing catheter inserted through the biopsy channel of the endoscope. The majority of highly dysplastic or malignant lesions remain unstained and clinical studies have shown that biopsy of these areas enhances detection of both high-grade dysplasia (HGD) and early squamous cell carcinoma [14,15,16]. The sensitivity for HGD or carcinoma ranges from 46 to 96% in published series [15,16], with differences in the sensitivity probably due to differing techniques and populations studied. Lugol's staining is also useful in estimating the extent of mucosal disease, which can be underestimated by endoscopy [17] and in differentiating regenerative squamous epithelium from small areas of residual Barrett's mucosa in patients who have undergone mucosal

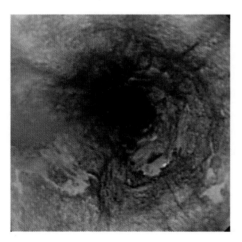

Figure 3.2 Lugol's iodine chromoendoscopy. Normal squamous epithelium is stained black, while the unstained areas reveal an extensive flat area of high-grade intraepithelial neoplasia (HGIN).

ablation. Lugol's staining is a straightforward technique, with unstained areas easy to identify. The technique does not require specialized equipment or additional staff, and there is a case to be made for its routine use in patients with epidemiological risk factors for SCC.

Methylene blue

Methylene blue is taken up by the cytoplasm of absorptive cells, such as goblet cells, which are present in Barrett's epithelium [18]. The technique used to stain the mucosa is more involved as the surface mucus must first be removed as it inhibits the uptake of methylene blue. A specialized spray catheter is used to spray 10% N-acetylcysteine over the mucosa using a volume of 3 ml/cm of Barrett's mucosa. Two minutes are allowed before a 0.5% solution of methylene blue dye is sprayed at a volume of 4 ml/cm of Barrett's mucosa. After a further 2 minutes the dye is vigorously washed away using 120–300 ml of water. This final wash is particularly important as insufficient irrigation results in incorrect staining and reduced sensitivity of targeted biopsy. Staining is deemed to be positive when the noneroded mucosa is stained blue despite vigorous irrigation [19]. Dysplastic change is associated with a reduction in goblet cell numbers and an increasing nuclear to cytoplasm ratio proportional to the degree of dysplasia, and such tissues absorb methylene blue to a lesser extent than surrounding cells. Increasing grades of dysplasia may appear as heterogeneous or unstained areas, allowing targeted rather than random biopsies to be taken [20] and have been reported to improve the detection of HGIN in Barrett's esophagus [19,21,22]. Canto et al. demonstrated a significant improvement in the diagnosis of dysplasia or cancer with methylene blue (12 versus 6%, $p = 0.004$) [19]. However, these results have not always been replicated in other studies [23,24,25,26], with other groups unable to demonstrate a significant difference in detecting intestinal metaplasia or dysplasia using methylene blue–directed biopsies versus conventional biopsies [24]. A recent randomized prospective crossover study that compared four-quadrant biopsies every 2 cm with methylene blue–directed biopsies demonstrated dysplasia in 17 of 18 patients with random four-quadrant biopsies compared with 9 of 18 in methylene–blue directed biopsies [27]. These results may be due to different staining techniques or related to a learning curve for the staining technique. One group has also raised concerns about possible induction of genetic damage by methylene blue [28]. Unlike Lugol's iodine, applying methylene blue is time-consuming and requires special equipment and additional staff, and at

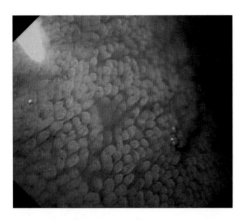

Figure 3.3 Indigo carmine chromoendoscopy combined with magnification in a patient with Barrett's oesophagus. The villiform but regular surface pattern, typical of Barrett's esophagus, can be appreciated. Biopsies showed no evidence of dysplasia.

present the generalizability of methylene blue staining to standard endoscopic practice remains unclear.

Indigo carmine

Indigo carmine is an alternative contrast-enhancing agent to methylene blue. Unlike Lugol's iodine or methylene blue, indigo carmine is not taken up by tissues but instead pools in crevices between epithelial cells, thereby highlighting small lesions or irregularities in the mucosal architecture (Figure 3.3). The dye is diluted to a 0.1–0.5% solution and sprayed directly onto the mucosa. While it has been extensively used to detect dysplasia and flat lesions during colonoscopy [29,30,31], there are relatively little data relating to esophageal cancer. In combination with magnification endoscopy (see p. 34), it may be useful in differentiating HGIN from nondysplastic Barrett's [32].

Outstanding issues with chromoendoscopy include the lack of uniformity in the method, concentration of the stain, and classification of staining patterns, making it difficult to compare reported studies.

Narrow band imaging

Narrow band imaging (NBI) uses filter systems that only allow the passage of those spectral components of light that are absorbed by mucosal blood vessels and hemoglobin. The surrounding mucosa reflects this light, and because of this, a maximum contrast of vessels and surrounding mucosa can be observed. In addition, the use of blue light, which has a shorter wavelength, means that only superficial structures are seen due to its shallow penetration depth and decreased optical

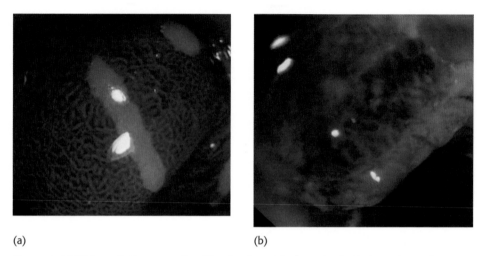

(a)   (b)

Figure 3.4 (a) High-resolution narrow band imaging (HR-NBI) of nondysplastic Barrett's esophagus. The regular villous (type 3) crypt pattern can easily be identified. (b) NBI of early cancer to compare with the normal pattern in (a).

scattering (Figure 3.4). As a consequence, the visualization of the capillary system is less distorted compared with white-light endoscopy and more surface detail is evident [33].

NBI has been shown to be superior in visualizing the columnar-lined epithelium and in visualizing Barrett's epithelium than standard endoscopy [34]. One group has found that a ridge/villous pattern and distorted pattern seen at NBI have a high correlation with intestinal metaplasia (*k* score of 0.79) and HGD (*k* score 0.97) [35], whilst Kara *et al.* [36] demonstrated that the addition of NBI or chromoendoscopy to high-resolution endoscopy increased the detection of HGD or early cancers from 79 to 86% and 93%, respectively, although this was not statistically significant. These studies are encouraging; however, an accepted classification system of mucosal or vascular patterns is required, and larger, prospective studies comparing NBI with other imaging techniques are needed.

Magnification endoscopy

Magnification endoscopes contain a movable lens at the distal tip for adjusting the focus and are able to magnify an image from 1.5× to 150× (Figures 3.5 and 3.6). Precise tip control is required to avoid blurring of the image, and a cap is often fitted to the distal tip of the endoscope, allowing the mucosa in contact with the cap to be magnified without the motility of the esophagus affecting visualization.

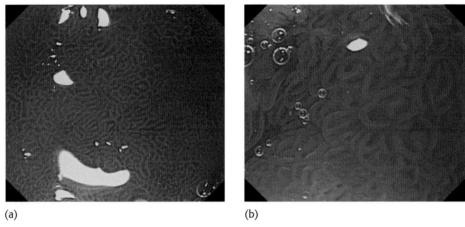

(a)   (b)

Figure 3.5 (a) Magnification endoscopy in a patient with Barrett's esophagus confirms a regular mucosal crypt pattern with no features suggestive of dysplasia (confirmed on biopsy). (b) Early superficial (5mm) adenocarcinoma arising in short-segment Barrett's esophagus just above the esophagogastric junction.

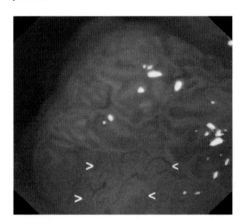

Figure 3.6 Magnification endoscopy in a patient with early cancer arising in Barrett's esophagus. The regular mucosal crypt pattern can be seen in the upper half of the image, but this pattern is distorted with short, corkscrew irregular blood vessels in the lower part of the figure (arrows) consistent with cancer, confirmed on biopsy.

Endoscopy is performed as usual, and when an area of interest is seen, a rotary dial on the control head of the instrument or a thumb-operated lever are used to zoom in and out of the endoscopic view [37].

Magnification endoscopy has been shown to be useful in identifying Barrett's esophagus [32]. In terms of early esophageal cancer, characteristic changes in the superficial microvascular architecture according to the depth of tumor invasion have been reported, with 83.3% agreement between histologic depth of invasion and magnification appearance [38]. Despite these promising results, magnification endoscopy is not widely used. One reason for this is that endoscopy time is prolonged up to 24 min, and varying results have been demonstrated from different studies that examined interobserver reproducibility, with kappa values results varying from <0.4 to 0.74 [26,39,40,41]. A uniform classification system for staining and magnification patterns does not yet exist, and varying sensitivity and specificity have been reported in detecting intestinal metaplasia and dysplasia [32,42,43,44]. Some of these variations may relate to the learning curve required for this technique, but the utility of magnification endoscopy in daily practice remains to be clarified.

Confocal endomicroscopy

Confocal endomicroscopy is a new tool that complements conventional white-light endoscopy. Where standard endoscopy images the mucosal surface with relatively low resolution over a large field of view, confocal microscopy allows visualization below the tissue surface, with subcellular resolution over a much smaller region of tissue. This is achieved by an adaptation of light microscopy that uses focal laser illumination of tissue planes by an optical fiber, which then detects only "in-focus" light through a pinhole and rejects "out-of-focus" light to provide a clear image from one focal plane [45,46]. Once an area of interest is visualized, so-called optical biopsies can be taken. This is a nondestructive, *in situ*, method of performing instantaneous mucosal histopathology without the risk of bleeding [47]. The addition of topical (acriflavine) or intravenous (fluorescein sodium) contrast agents provides further details about cellular architecture. Kiesslich *et al.* [48] demonstrated a sensitivity and specificity for detecting Barrett's esophagus of 98.8 and 94.4%, respectively, and for associated neoplasia of 91.7 and 99.0%, respectively, giving an accuracy of 97.5% in 42 patients with good interobserver agreement (k 0.84) [49]. Image acquisition time and time taken to assess potentially large surface area are concerns but may be offset by the need to take fewer biopsies. Further studies are required to confirm these promising preliminary results and to clarify the exact role of confocal endomicroscopy in screening for and staging esophageal cancer.

Optical coherence tomography

Optical coherence tomography (OCT) is an emerging endoscopic technique, which provides a cross-sectional, subsurface imaging of the gastrointestinal tract. OCT is similar in principle to ultrasonography but uses light waves rather than acoustic waves, using the back-reflection of infrared light from the mucosal layers of the gut to form an image of the mucosa and submucosa. OCT is performed using a catheter probe introduced through the instrument biopsy channel, and scanning probes are available to create either radial or linear images. These provide a resolution to within 7–20 μm with a scanning depth of 1–2 mm. This level of resolution allows visualization of the mucosal glands, crypts, and villi but does not allow visualization of cellular features such as nuclear abnormalities in dysplasia. Color Doppler has been used in an experimental setting that allows visualization of subsurface blood vessels [49].

The normal layers of the esophagus from the epithelium to the muscularis propria can be seen [50,51,52,53]. These layers are disrupted in Barrett's esophagus, with preliminary results comparing normal oesophagus, Barrett's, and normal stomach demonstrating excellent sensitivity of 97% and specificity of 92% [54]. A study by Evans et al. [55] examined the potential of OCT to differentiate intramucosal carcinoma (IMC) and HGD from specialized intestinal metaplasia, indeterminate-grade dysplasia, and low-grade dysplasia (LGD). They found that there was a significant relationship between histopathologic diagnosis of IMC/HGD and image features. When three or more image features were present, the sensitivity and specificity for diagnosing IMC/HGD was 83 and 75%, respectively.

A further development is spectroscopic OCT. This uses the broad spectral bandwidth of the optical source to obtain information from the spectral content of the backscattered light. Spectral OCT has been compared with regular OCT in Barrett's esophagus and has been shown to improve the contrast of the images [50]. It is currently too early to define what role, if any, OCT will play in the diagnosis or staging of patients with upper gastrointestinal malignancy.

Autofluorescence imaging

Autofluorescence imaging (AFI) endoscopy involves stimulation of certain endogenous molecules (fluorophores) by ultraviolet or blue light. On excitation, these fluorophores emit fluorescent light spread over a range of longer wavelengths in the green to red spectrum. This is called autofluorescence, and responsible endogenous fluorophores include collagen, reduced nicotinamide adenine dinucleotide, aromatic amino acids, and porphyrins (Figure 3.7). AFI endoscopy can detect HGD and early cancer in Barrett's esophagus [56]. Two randomized controlled trials have examined the role of AFI in diagnosing esophageal adenocarcinoma. Borovicka et al. found one additional neoplastic lesion for every 21 patients examined [57]. However, a study by Kara et al. was unable to demonstrate a difference in detecting HGD and esophageal adenocarcinoma between AFI and

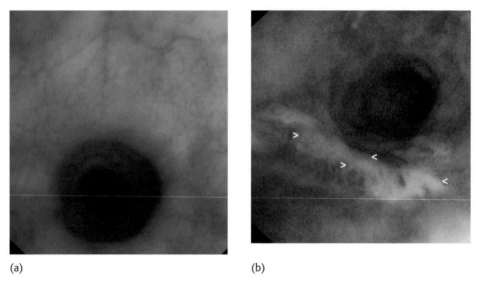

(a)   (b)

Figure 3.7 (a) Normal green mucosal appearance in autofluorescence (AFI) imaging. (b) Early carcinoma is seen as a pink/magenta area (arrows) using autofluorescence.

conventional endoscopy [58]. Both these studies had high false-positive rates of 78 and 87%, respectively; however, both these studies used an older AFI system capturing information from reflected light using fiberoptic endoscopes with low-quality images. Using a newer videoendoscopic AFI system, it has been possible to identify HGD or early cancer in 6 of 21 patients with Barrett's esophagus that was not identified using conventional endoscopy [59]. Again there was a high false-positive rate of 50%. The authors therefore compared the performance of AFI in combination with NBI in 20 patients with Barrett's esophagus and suspected or confirmed HGIN [60]. AFI identified 47 suspicious lesions, of which 28 had HGIN and 19 (40%) were false positive. In these latter 19 cases, the use of NBI correctly identified 14 as nondysplastic, reducing the overall false-positive rate to 10%. This study suggests that combining AFI and NBI may increase the accuracy of detecting HGIN in Barrett's esophagus. Larger, controlled studies are awaited and refinements in technology may further improve these impressive early results.

Other modalities

A number of other endoscopic modalities have shown promise in the detection of early neoplasia. In *Raman spectroscopy*, light can be absorbed or scattered as it interacts with tissue molecules. Almost all of the scattered light is the same wavelength as the incidence light; however, a small fraction undergoes Raman scattering, in which slight shifts in energy and wavelength occur because of exchange of energy with the molecular structure. These wavelength shifts correspond to specific vibrations of the interacting molecule. A Raman spectrum is a plot of the intensity of the scattered light as a function of the wavelength shift, with each peak corresponding to a specific molecular state. Characteristic plots for normal tissue can be developed, allowing abnormal spectra to be easily identified. One group has demonstrated an accuracy of 88% for differentiating dysplastic or early malignant change from nondysplastic tissue in 100 patients with Barrett's esophagus [61].

Elastic scatter spectroscopy also shows promise in the detection of early cancer. In a study by Lovat *et al.*, elastic scattering spectroscopy detected HGD or cancer with 92% sensitivity and 60% specificity, and differentiated HGD and cancer from inflammation with a sensitivity and specificity of 79%. Using this technique, the authors calculated that the number of biopsies of nondysplastic or low-grade dysplasia could be decreased by 60% with minimal loss of accuracy, while negative spectroscopy results would exclude HGD or cancer with an accuracy greater than 99.5%. These preliminary results are promising, but corroborating studies are awaited.

Wireless capsule endoscopy (WCE), now a cornerstone of gastroenterological practice in investigating small bowel disease, may have a potential role to play in early cancer detection. WCE consists of a video imaging chip, illuminating diode system, two batteries, and a radio transmitter that transmits data to an external receiver. There are several factors that make it an appealing option, including its small size (26×11 mm), noninvasive nature, and the fact that it could be performed in a primary care setting. Initial studies examining its role in the upper gastrointestinal tract have shown that it is effective in detecting esophageal varices and portal hypertensive gastropathy in a high-prevalence population [62]. In another study, WCE correctly identified all patients with both short- and long-segment Barrett's esophagus [63]. The inability to take biopsies is a limitation that needs to be overcomed, and at present, it is unclear what role WCE may play in esophageal cancer diagnosis.

Conclusion

Endoscopy is evolving rapidly, allowing increasingly accurate assessment of mucosal appearances, especially Barrett's esophagus and early neoplasia, hopefully allowing a more targeted approach and selective approach to biopsy practice.

Large, controlled, prospective studies examining the different novel endoscopic modalities are required to clarify which if any will predominate and enter routine clinical practice.

REFERENCES

1. C. Donnelan, D. Forman, and S. Everett. The epidemiology of upper gastrointestinal malignancies: current perspectives and projections of disease burden. In *The Effective Management of Upper Gastrointestinal Malignancies*, eds. D. Cunningham, J. Jankowski, and A. Miles. (London: Aesculapius Medical Press, 2005), 3–21.
2. W. Blot, S. S. Devesa, R. W. Kneller, *et al.* Rising incidence of adenocarcinoma of the esophagus and gastric cardia. *JAMA*, **165** (1991), 1287–9.
3. M. Pera, A. J. Cameron, V. F. Trasteck, *et al.* Increasing incidence of adenocarcinoma of the esophagus and esophagogastric junction. *Gastroenterology*, **104** (1993), 510–3.
4. A. Newnham, M. J. Quinn, P. Babb, *et al.* Trends in oesophageal and gastric cancer incidence, mortality and survival in England and Wales 1971–1998/1999. *Aliment Pharmacol Ther*, **17** (2003), 655–64.
5. Medical Research Council (MRC). Surgical resection with or without preoperative chemotherapy in oesophageal cancer: a randomised controlled trial. *Lancet*, **359**:9319 (2002), 1727–33.
6. F. Fiorica, D. De Bona, F. Schepis, *et al.* Preoperative chemoradiotherapy for oesophageal cancer: a systematic review and meta-analysis. *Gut*, **53** (2004), 925–30.
7. C. P. Dooley, A. W. Larson, N. H. Stace, *et al.* Double contrast barium meal and upper gastrointestinal endoscopy. A comparative study. *Ann Intern Med*, **101** (1984), 538–45.
8. J. O'Donoghue, R. Waldron, D. Gough, *et al.* An analysis of the diagnostic accuracy of endoscopic biopsy and cytology in the detection of oesophageal malignancy. *Eur J Surg Oncol*, **18** (1992), 332–4.
9. D. Faigel, C. Deveney, D. Phillips, *et al.* Biopsy-negative malignant esophageal stricture: diagnosis by endoscopic ultrasound. *Am J Gastroenterol*, **93** (1998), 2257–60.
10. J. Siewert and H. J. Stein. Classification of adenocarcinoma of the oesophagogastric junction. *Br J Surg*, **85** (1998), 1457–9.
11. Japanese Society for Esophageal Diseases. *Guidelines for the Clinical and Pathological Studies on Carcinoma of the Esophagus*, 9th edn. (Tokyo: Kanehara, 1999).
12. Participants in the Paris Workshop. The Paris endoscopic classification of superficial neoplastic lesions: esophagus, stomach, and colon: November 30 to December 1, 2002. *Gastrointest Endosc*, **58**:Suppl. (2003), S3–43.
13. K. Sugimachi, K. Kitamura, K. Baba, *et al.* Endoscopic diagnosis of early carcinoma of the esophagus using Lugol's solution. *Gastrointest Endosc*, **38** (1992), 657–61.
14. A. Yokoyama, T. Ohmori, H. Makuuchi, *et al.* Successful screening for early esophageal cancer in alcoholics using endoscopy and mucosa iodine staining. *Cancer*, **76** (1995), 919–21.

15. S. Dawsey, D. E. Fleischer, G. Q. Wang, *et al.* Mucosal iodine staining improves endoscopic visualization of squamous dysplasia and squamous cell carcinoma of the esophagus in Linxian, China. *Cancer*, **83** (1998), 220–31.

16. R. Fagundes, S. G. S. de Barros, A. C. K. Putten, *et al.* Occult dysplasia is disclosed by Lugol chromoendoscopy in alcoholics at high risk for squamous cell carcinoma of the esophagus. *Endoscopy*, **31** (1999), 281–5.

17. V. Meyer, P. Burtin, B. Bour, *et al.* Endoscopic detection of early esophageal cancer in a high-risk population: does Lugol staining improve videoendoscopy? *Gastrointest Endosc*, **45** (1997), 480–4.

18. D. Carr-Locke, F. H. Al-Chaws, M. S. Branch, *et al.* Technology assessment status evaluation: endoscopic tissue staining and tattooing. *Gastrointest Endosc*, **43** (1996), 652–6.

19. M. Canto, S. Setrakian, J. Willis, *et al.* Methylene blue directed biopsies improve detection of intestinal metaplasia and dysplasia in Barrett's esophagus. *Gastrointest Endosc*, **51** (2000), 560–8.

20. M. Canto, S. Setrakian, J. Willis, *et al.* Methylene blue staining of dysplastic and non-dysplastic Barrett's esophagus: an in vivo and ex vivo study. *Endoscopy*, **33** (2001), 391–400.

21. M. Canto, T. Yoshida, and L. Gossner. Chromoscopy of intestinal metaplasia in Barrett's esophagus. *Endoscopy*, **34** (2002), 330–6.

22. R. Kiesslich, M. F. Neurath, and P. R. Galle. Chromoendoscopy and magnifying endoscopy in patients with gastrooesophageal reflux disease. Useful or negligible? *Dig Dis*, **22** (2004), 142–7.

23. R. Wong, J. Horwhat, and C. Maydonovitch. Sky blue or murky waters: the diagnostic utility of methylene blue. *Gastrointest Endosc*, **54** (2001), 409–13.

24. J. Wo, M. B. Ray, S. Mayfield-Stokes, *et al.* Comparison of methylene blue-directed biopsies and conventional biopsies in the detection of intestinal metasplasia and dysplasia in Barrett's esophagus: a preliminary study. *Gastroinest Endosc*, **54** (2001), 294–301.

25. K. Egger, M. Werner, A. Meining, *et al.* Biopsy surveillance is still necessary in patients with Barrett's oesophagus despite new endoscopic imaging techniques. *Gut*, **52** (2003), 18–23.

26. A. Meining, T. Rosche, R. Kiesslich, *et al.* Inter- and intra-observer variability of magnification chromoendoscopy for detecting specialized intestinal metaplasia at the gastroesophageal junction. *Endoscopy*, **36** (2004), 160–4.

27. CH. Lim, Rotimi, O., Dexter, SPL. *et al.* Randomized crossover study that used methylene blue or random 4-quadrant biopsy for the diagnosis of dysplasia in Barrett's esophagus. *Gastrointestinal Endoscopy*, **64** (2006), 195–99.

28. J. Olliver, C. P. Wild, P. Sahay, *et al.* Chromoendoscopy with methylene blue and associated DNA damage in Barrett's oesophagus. *Lancet*, **362** (2003), 373–4.

29. E. Jaramillo, M. Watanabe, P. Slezak, *et al.* Flat neoplastic lesions of the colon and rectum detected by high-resolution video endoscopy and chromoscopy. *Gastrointest Endosc*, **42** (1995), 114–22.

30. R. Kiesslich, M. von Bergh, M. Hahn, *et al.* Chromoendoscopy with indigocarmine improves the detection of adenomatous and nonadenomatous lesions in the colon. *Endoscopy*, **33** (2001), 1001–6.

31. J. C. Brooker, B. P. Saunders, S. G. Shah, *et al.* Total colonic dye-spray increases the detection of diminutive adenomas during routine colonoscopy: a randomised controlled trial. *Gastrointest Endosc*, **56** (2002), 333–8.

32. P. Sharma, A. P. Weston, M. Topalovski, *et al.* Magnification chromoendoscopy for the detection of intestinal metaplasia and dysplasia in Barrett's oesophagus. *Gut,* **52** (2003), 24–7.

33. H. Messemann and A. Probst. Narrow band imaging in Barrett's esophagus- where are we standing? *Gastrointest Endosc,* **65** (2007), 47–9.

34. Y. Hammamoto, T. Endo, K. Nosho, *et al.* Usefulness of narrow-band imaging endoscopy for diagnosis of Barrett's esophagus. *J Gastroenterol,* **39** (2004), 14–20.

35. P. Sharma, A. Bansal, S. Mathur, *et al.* The utility of a novel narrow band imaging endoscopy system in patients with Barrett's esophagus. *Gastroinest Endosc,* **64** (2006), 167–75.

36. M. Kara, F. P. Peters, W. G. Rosmolen, *et al.* High-resolution endoscopy plus chromoendoscopy or narrow-band imaging in Barrett's esophagus: a prospective randomised crossover study. *Endoscopy,* **37** (2005), 929–36.

37. P. Sharma. Magnification endoscopy. *Gastrointest Endosc,* **61** (2005), 435–43.

38. Y. Kumagai, H. Inoue, K. Nagai, *et al.* Magnifying endoscopy, steroscopic microscopy and the microvascular architecture of superficial esophageal carcinoma. *Endoscopy,* **34** (2002), 269–375.

39. M. Dinis-Ribeiro, A. Costa-Pereira, C. Lopes, *et al.* Magnification chromoendoscopy for the diagnosis of gastric intestinal metaplasia and dysplasia. *Gastrointest Endosc,* **57** (2003), 498–504.

40. B. Mayinger, Y. Oezturk, M. Stolte, *et al.* Evaluation of sensitivity and inter- and intra-observer variability in the detection of intestinal metaplasia and dysplasia in Barrett's esophagus with enhanced magnification endoscopy. *Scand J Gastroenterol,* **41** (2006), 349–56.

41. P. Fortun, G. K. Anagnostopoulos, P. Kaye, *et al.* Acetic acid-enhanced magnification endoscopy in the diagnosis of specialized intestinal metaplasia, dysplasia and early cancer in Barrett's oesophagus. *Aliment Pharmacol Ther,* **23** (2006), 735–42.

42. K. Yagi, A. Nakamura, and A. Sekine. Accuracy of magnifying endoscopy with methylene blue in the diagnosis of specialized intestinal metaplasia and short-segment Barrett's esophagus in Japanese patients without *Helicobacter pylori* infection. *Gastrointest Endosc,* **58** (2003), 189–95.

43. H. Toyoda, C. Rubio, R. Befrits, *et al.* Detection of intestinal metaplasia in distal esophagus and esophagogastric junction by enhanced-magnification endoscopy. *Gastrointest Endosc,* **59** (2004), 15–21.

44. T. Endo, T. Awakawa, H. Takahashi, *et al.* Classification of Barrett's epithelium by magnifying endoscopy. *Gastrointest Endosc,* **55** (2002), 641–7.

45. J. Poneros. Optical coherence tomography and the detection of dysplasia in Barrett's esophagus. *Gastrointest Endosc,* **62** (2005), 832–3.

46. R. Kiesslich, J. Burgh, M. Vieth, *et al.* Confocal laser endoscopy for diagnosing intraepithelial neoplasias and colorectal cancer in vivo. *Gastroenterology,* **127** (2004), 706–13.

47. A. Polgase, W. J. McLaren, S. A. Skinner, *et al.* A fluorescence confocal endomicroscope for in vivo microscopy of the upper- and the lower-GI tract. *Gastrointest Endosc,* **62** (2005), 686–95.

48. R. Kiesslich, A. Dahlmann, M. Vieth, *et al.* In vivo histology of Barrett's esophagus and associated neoplasias by confocal laser endomicroscopy (abstract). *Gastrointest Endosc,* **61** (2005), AB101.

49. R. Wong, S. Yazdanfar, J. A. Izatt, *et al.* Visualization of subsurface blood vessels by color Doppler optical coherence tomography in rats: before and after hemostatic therapy. *Gastrointest Endosc*, **55** (2002), 88–95.

50. X. Li, S. A. Boppart, J. Van Dam, *et al.* Optical coherence tomography: advanced technology for the endoscopic imaging of Barrett's esophagus. *Endoscopy*, **32** (2000), 921–30.

51. K. Kobayashi, J. A. Izatt, M. D. Kulkarni, *et al.* High-resolution cross-sectional imaging of the gastrointestinal tract using optical coherence tomography: preliminary results. *Gastrointest Endosc*, **47** (1998), 515–23.

52. B. Bouma, G. J. Tearney, C. C. Compton, *et al.* High-resolution imaging of the human esophagus and stomach in vivo using optical coherence tomography. *Gastrointest Endosc*, **51** (2000), 467–74.

53. M. Sivak, K. Kobayashi, J. A. Izatt, *et al.* High-resolution endoscopic imaging of the GI tract using optical coherence tomography. *Gastrointest Endosc*, **51** (2000), 474–9.

54. J. Poneros, S. Brand, B. E. Bouma, *et al.* Diagnosis of specialized intestinal metaplasia by optical coherence tomography. *Gastroenterology*, **120** (2001), 7–12.

55. J. A. Evans, J. M. Poneros, B. E. Bouma, *et al.* Optical coherence tomography to identify intramucosal carcinoma and high-grade dysplasia in Barrett's esophagus. *Clin Gastroenterol Hepatol*, **4**:1 (2006), 38–43.

56. J. Haringsma, G. N. Tygat, H. Yano, *et al.* Autofluorescence endoscopy feasibility of detection of GI neoplasma unapparent to while light endoscopy with an evolving technology. *Gastrointest Endosc*, **53** (2001), 642–50.

57. J. Borovicka, J. Fischer, J. Neuweiler, *et al.* Role of autofluorescence endoscopy in surveillance of Barrett's esophagus: a prospective multicenter randomised trial (abstract). *Gastrointest Endosc*, **61** (2005), AB103.

58. M. Kara, M. E. Smiths, W. E. Rosmolen, *et al.* A randomised crossover study comparing light-induced fluorescence endoscopy with standard videoendoscopy for detection of early neoplasia in Barrett's esophagus. *Gastrointest Endosc*, **61** (2005), 671–8.

59. M. Kara, F. P. Peters, F. J. Ten Kate, *et al.* Endoscopic video autofluorescence imaging may improve the detection of early neoplasia in patients with Barrett's esophagus. *Gastrointest Endosc*, **61** (2005), 679–85.

60. M. Kara, F. P. Peters, P. Fockens, *et al.* Endoscopic video-autofluorescence imaging followed by narrow band imaging for detecting early neoplasia in Barrett's esophagus. *Gastrointest Endosc*, **64** (2006), 176–85.

61. L.-M. W. K. Song, A. Molckovsky, K. Wang, *et al.* Diagnostic accuracy of Raman spectroscopy for the classification of dysplastic lesions in Barrett's esophagus (abstract). *Gastrointest Endosc*, **63** (2006), AB89.

62. G. Eisen, R. Eliakim, A. Zaman, *et al.* The accuracy of PillCam ESO capsule endoscopy versus conventional upper endoscopy for the diagnosis of esophageal varices: a prospective three-centre pilot study. *Endoscopy*, **38** (2006), 31–5.

63. F. C. Ramirez, M. S. Shaukat, M. A. Young, *et al.* Feasibility and safety of string, wireless capsule endoscopy in the diagnosis of Barrett's esophagus. *Hepatology*, **19** (2004), 433–9.

4

Endoscopic Ultrasound in Esophageal Cancer

Anne Marie Lennon and Ian D. Penman

Introduction

The major role for endoscopic ultrasound (EUS) is in defining stage of disease. Tumors are staged using the TNM classification, which describes the anatomic extent of cancer at the time of diagnosis and before therapy (Table 4.1) [1]. This allows a classification of the stages of cancer for estimation of prognosis and comparing the results of different treatments (Table 4.2). The definitions of TNM are based on the depth of invasion of the tumor into the esophageal wall or beyond (T stage), the presence or absence of regional lymph node involvement (N stage), and identification of distant metastasis (M stage). EUS provides uniquely detailed images of the different layers of the esophagus and surrounding structures. Using standard EUS (5–12 MHz), the esophageal wall is visualized as five layers that correspond to the mucosa (layers 1 and 2), submucosa (layer 3), muscularis propria (layer 4), and the outer, adventitial layer (layer 5) (Figure 4.1).

T staging

Tis is the earliest stage, defined as tumor present in the epithelium but not invading the lamina propria. T1 tumors involve the lamina propria and the submucosa. These can be further subclassified as T1 m where the tumor is confined to the mucosa and T1sm where the tumor invades the submucosa (Figure 4.2). Tumors that invade the muscularis propria are classified as T2 (Figure 4.3), while tumors involving the adventitia are termed T3 (Figure 4.4). Involvement of mediastinal structures such as the pleura, azygous vein, aorta, or adjacent structures indicates T4 disease (Figure 4.5).

EUS is the most accurate method of determining T stage and has been shown consistently to outperform computer tomography (CT) for locoregional staging of

Carcinoma of the Esophagus, ed. Sheila C. Rankin. Published by Cambridge University Press. © Cambridge University Press 2008.

Table 4.1 TNM staging system for esophageal cancer [1]

Stage	Definition
TX	Primary tumor cannot be assessed
T0	No evidence of primary tumor
Tis	Carcinoma *in situ*
T1	Tumor invades lamina propria and submucosa
T2	Tumor invades muscularis propria
T3	Tumor invades adventitia
T4	Tumor invades adjacent structures
NX	Regional lymph nodes cannot be assessed
N0	No regional lymph node metastases
N1	Regional lymph node metastases
MX	Distant metastases cannot be assessed
M0	No distant metastases
M1a	Coeliac nodes involved in lower esophageal cancer
	Cervical nodes involved in upper esophageal cancer*
M1b	Beyond locoregional node involvement, i.e., celiac nodes in upper esophageal cancer
	Metastatic involvement of visceral organs, pleura, peritoneum
	Nonregional lymph nodes and/or other distant metastases

*For tumors of the midthoracic esophagus, M1a is not applicable.

Table 4.2 Staging of esophageal cancer [1]

	T	N	M
Stage 0	Tis	N0	M0
Stage I	T1	N0	M0
Stage IIA	T2	N0	M0
	T3	N0	M0
Stage IIB	T1	N1	M0
	T2	N1	M0
Stage III	T3	N1	M0
	T4	Any N	M0
Stage IV	Any T	Any N	M1
Stage IVA	Any T	Any N	M1a
Stage IVB	Any T	Any N	M1b

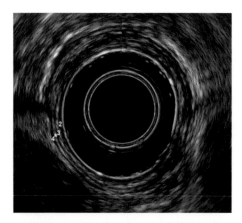

Figure 4.1 Electronic radial EUS (10 MHz) image showing the normal 5 layer pattern of the esophageal wall. The first layer (rarely seen) represents the fluid-tissue interface, the hypoechoic (black) second layer (2) is the mucosa, the third layer is the submucosal (3), seen as a hyperechoic (white) band. The muscularis propria is usually seen as a single hypoechoic outer layer (4), but here the high resolution near field imaging is able to distinguish the inner and outer layer of the muscularis with the fibrous hyperechoic band separating them (*).

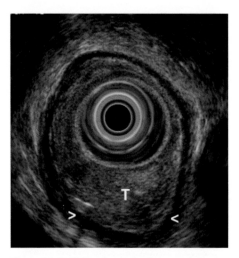

Figure 4.2 Radial endoscopic ultrasound (EUS) image of T1 carcinoma (T). Although bulky, the lesion is confined to the mucosa and submucosa and does not invade into the muscularis propria (arrows).

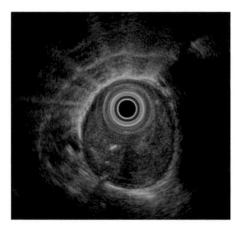

Figure 4.3 T2 carcinoma.

esophageal cancer [2,3,4,5]. In a meta-analysis, Rosch et al. found that EUS had an accuracy for T stage of 85–90% compared with 50–80% for CT [3]. A more recent meta-analysis by Lightdale and Kulkarni [5] found a similar accuracy of 80% for all T stages that increased to 90% for T3 lesions.

Accurate staging of early esophageal cancers (T1) is important, as T1 m tumors are associated with a low risk of nodal involvement compared with T1sm lesions that are associated with nodal positivity in up to 25% of cases [6,7]. This

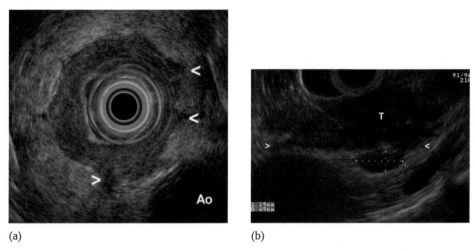

(a)   (b)

Figure 4.4 (a) Bulky T3 carcinoma. The tumor has invaded through the muscularis propria into the perioesophageal fat but does not invade the aorta (Ao, bottom right). (b) Linear endoscopic ultrasound (EUS) image showing a large tumor (T) invading through the muscularis propria (arrows) with an irregular outer margin and a 12 × 5 mm peritumoral lymph node.

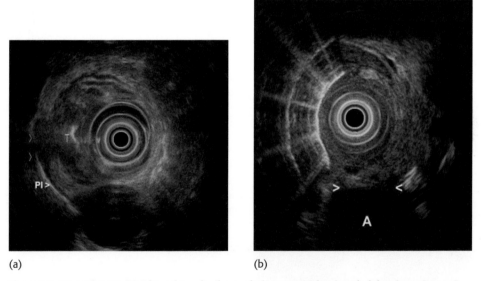

(a)   (b)

Figure 4.5   T4 carcinoma. (a) A large irregular, hypoechoic tumor (T) has invaded the pleura (arrows). (b) The tumor is adherent to the anterior surface of the aorta (A) with loss of the normal echorich plane of separation (arrows).

differentiation is crucial, as it allows the identification of those who may be suitable for local therapy such as endoscopic mucosal resection (EMR) [8]. Standard EUS, which uses frequencies of 5–12 MHz, is however limited in its ability to make this important distinction [3,9,10]. High-frequency catheter probes (HFCPs) have been developed with imaging frequencies from 15 to 30 MHz. These small-diameter, nonoptic probes are passed through the working channel of a standard endoscope. The higher frequency allows greater definition of esophageal wall layers at the expense of depth of penetration (average 2.9 cm). Using these HFCPs, the esophagus is viewed as a nine-layer structure, with layers 1 and 2 representing the epithelium, layer 3 the lamina propria, layer 4 the muscularis mucosa, layer 5 the submucosa, layer 6 the circular muscle layer, layer 7 the connective tissue, layer 8 the longitudinal muscle, and layer 9 the adventitia (Figure 4.6). HFCPs have shown promise in identifying early esophageal cancer with accuracies of 87–92% reported compared with 62–76% for standard EUS [11,12]. Other studies of HFCPs report accuracies of between 65 and 100% [11,13,14,15,16,17,18,19,20], but many of these contain small numbers of patients. HFCPs have poor depth of penetration and so not surprisingly have a lower sensitivity for detecting nodal involvement, 56% compared with 82% for standard EUS in one study [21]. Thus, if HFCPs are used, standard EUS should be performed as well to assess for nodal and metastatic disease. Other problems associated with HFCPs include the need to instill water in the lumen (unless a balloon sheath is used), which may increase the risk of aspiration. Although HFCPs are reusable, they are expensive, have a limited lifetime, and undergo image deterioration with repeated use.

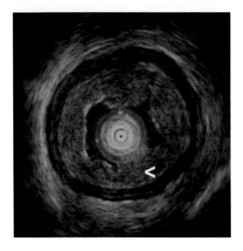

Figure 4.6 High-frequency catheter probe endoscopic ultrasound (EUS; 12 MHz). In a patient with early esophageal cancer the circumferential tumor invades the submucosa (T1sm, arrow), but there is no involvement of the muscularis propria.

N staging

Esophageal cancer is associated with a high incidence of nodal disease, with 60% of T2 and over 80% of T3 or T4 tumors node positive [22]. The presence of an increasing number of malignant nodes is associated with a worse outcome with reported 5-year survival rates for 0, 1–3, 4–7, and 8 or more involved lymph nodes of 53.3, 33.8, 17, and 0%, respectively [23]. Other authors have demonstrated that patients with greater than four involved regional lymph nodes have a particularly poor outcome [24]. Although the presence of nodal disease does not preclude successful tumor resection, it is associated with cure rates after surgery of only 5–10% [22,23,25,26], highlighting the importance of accurate detection of nodal involvement so that such patients can be considered for neoadjuvant therapy [27].

Both benign and malignant lymph nodes can be seen by EUS. Endoscopic features suggestive of malignancy include a short-axis diameter greater than 5 mm, a round shape, distinct outer border, and hypoechoity (Figure 4.7) [28,29]. The presence of all four features is associated with 80% accuracy for malignant involvement [29]. Based on these features, meta-analyses have shown the accuracy of EUS for N staging of 75–79% [3,30]. Studies comparing EUS and CT for the evaluation of regional lymph node staging have consistently demonstrated that endoscopic ultrasound is more accurate [3,4,31,32,33,34]. Studies comparing ^{18}F-fluoro-deoxy-D-glucose-positron emission tomography (FDG-PET) with EUS for local node staging show that FDG-PET has a lower sensitivity (32–37 versus 81–89%) but a higher specificity (89–100 versus 54–67%) compared with EUS [35,36,37].

Although the presence of all four endoscopic features is highly accurate at predicting malignant involvement, all four criteria are found in only 25% of

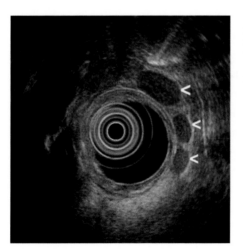

Figure 4.7 N1 lymph node status. Several periesophageal lymph nodes with endosonographic features suspicious of malignancy are present (size, shape, discrete border, and hypoechoity).

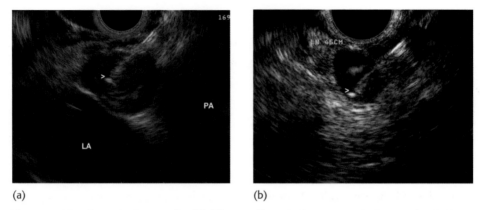

(a)   (b)

Figure 4.8 (a) Endoscopic ultrasound–guided fine-needle aspiration (EUS-FNA). A 1-cm subcarinal lymph node with features suspicious for malignancy is targeted for FNA. The needle tip can be clearly seen within the lymph node (arrow). LA, left atrium; PA, pulmonary artery. (b) EUS-FNA of a 6-mm left gastric artery lymph node (LN). Cytology confirmed adenocarcinoma.

malignant nodes [29]. Because of this, EUS-guided fine-needle aspiration (EUS-FNA) was developed to sample potentially malignant lymph nodes (Figure 4.8). EUS-FNA has been shown to increase accuracy compared with EUS alone. An example of this is by Vazquez-Sequeiros *et al.* who compared a historical cohort of 33 patients with 31 patients who underwent EUS-FNA of non peritumoral lymph nodes. Compared with EUS alone, EUS-FNA was associated with significantly better sensitivity (63 versus 93%) and accuracy (70 versus 93%) [6]. One problem with EUS-FNA is that it prolongs the procedure, while the need for an FNA needle increases the cost. Vazquez-Sequeiros *et al.* recently addressed this problem in a prospective study [38]. They compared the four classic lymph node criteria with the four classic criteria plus three additional criteria (celiac region lymph node; number of lymph nodes ≥ 5; or T3/4 tumor stage). All lymph nodes were then sampled and the modified EUS criteria were found to be more accurate than standard criteria (ROC 0.88 versus 0.78). The presence of six or more criteria was associated with 100% positive predictive value for N1 disease, while all those with no positive modified EUS criteria had N0 disease. The maximum accuracy (86%) was achieved when three or more of the seven modified criteria were present. Based on these results, it has been suggested that in patients with either ≥ 6 or 0 criterion, FNA may be avoided, as the results are unlikely to change the N stage. Using this approach, 42% of patients in this study could have avoided FNA, which was associated with a cost saving of $117.84 per patient. Further studies are required to confirm these data.

M staging

Involvement of tumor at sites distant from the primary tumor or distant lymph nodes is considered metastatic disease. In those with no evidence of metastatic disease on CT or FDG-PET, EUS is usually undertaken. EUS allows the visualization of the celiac axis and surrounding lymph nodes, the left lobe of the liver, and the adrenals. The most commonly used definition of celiac axis lymph nodes in the UK includes all nodes within 1 cm of the origin of the celiac trunk, while 2 cm is often used in the USA. This definition is, however, arbitrary, as it can sometimes be difficult to differentiate lymph nodes occurring along the left gastric artery from true celiac axis lymph nodes. EUS provides excellent imaging of the celiac lymph nodes (Figure 4.9), with an accuracy of 81–98% for detecting malignant involvement [31,39,40,41,42]. The mere presence of identifiable celiac lymph nodes is associated with a high incidence of malignant involvement, with one study finding that over 90% of celiac lymph nodes were malignant regardless of echo features or size, while 100% were malignant if they were greater than 1 cm [40]. A retrospective study by Romagnuolo *et al.* found that high-quality, thin-slice helical CT only detected 53% of celiac lymph nodes proven to be involved by EUS-FNA [43]. The left lobe of the liver should also be examined when staging an esophageal cancer. The medial two-third of the liver is well visualized with EUS with liver metastases found in 6.8% to 7% of patients with oesophageal cancer using EUS (Figure 4.10) [44,45], with 2.3% of these not detected on CT in one study [45]. When liver lesions are found, EUS-FNA can be used to confirm the diagnosis [46]. There are little data comparing EUS with multidetector CT, and it may be that EUS offers few advantages over multidetector CT in detecting liver involvement.

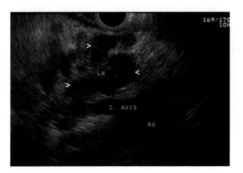

Figure 4.9 Linear endoscopic ultrasound (EUS) shows a poorly defined cluster of malignant-looking lymph nodes close to the origin of the celiac axes from aorta (Ao). Fine-needle aspiration (FNA) confirmed malignancy (Stage M1a).

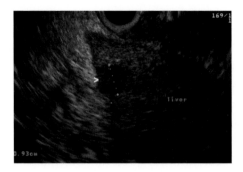

Figure 4.10 Linear endoscopic ultrasound (EUS) reveals a 9-mm hypoechoic lesion close to the surface of the left lobe of liver and fine-needle aspiration (FNA) confirmed adenocarcinoma.

EUS staging following neoadjuvant therapy

Neoadjuvant treatment aims to shrink the primary tumor and eradicate lymphatic and hematogenous micrometastases; however, neoadjuvant therapy is associated with toxicity and only 50% of patients respond to currently available regimens. Thus early detection of nonresponders may prevent unnecessary therapy associated toxicity and impact on treatment planning. Initial studies demonstrated accuracies of between 29 and 59% in terms of T and N staging probably due to the fact that EUS cannot differentiate fibrosis and inflammation associated with chemoradiotherapy from residual cancer within the esophageal wall [47,48,49,50,51]. Several studies have reported that a 50% or greater reduction in maximum cross-sectional area is relatively accurate at predicting response [52,53,54], while two studies have found an association between a measured reduction in cross-sectional area and survival [52,55]. Compared with other imaging modalities, CT was shown in a systematic review of the literature to have a significantly lower overall accuracy compared with EUS or FDG-PET, while EUS and FDG-PET had similar accuracies with maximum joint sensitivities of 86 and 85%, respectively [56].

Clinical impact of EUS

One group have examined the effect of EUS on outcome and reported that EUS is associated with a recurrence-free survival advantage and an overall survival advantage for patients [57]. The reason for this appears to be due an increase in the administration of chemoradiotherapy through more accurate preoperative staging. EUS has also been shown to alter patient management, increasing the number of referrals for nonsurgical palliation and decreasing cost [58,59,60]. EUS is cost-effective [61] with a study comparing CT, EUS-FNA, PET, and laparoscopy, demonstrating that CT in combination with EUS-FNA was the least expensive staging strategy [62].

Weaknesses of EUS staging

One of the major limitation of EUS staging is the inability to traverse a malignant stricture, which occurs in 20–30% of esophageal cancer patients (Figure 4.11) [63,64,65]. Early EUS studies showed a high incidence of perforation if EUS was performed after esophageal dilatation to 16–17 mm [63,66]; however, more recent studies have considerably lower perforation rates [65,67,68]. In a recent study of 132 patients with esophageal cancer, 32% required dilatation (14–16 mm) to complete the procedure, with only one perforation reported [67]. One reason for the differences in the rate of perforation in these two studies is that echoendoscopic technology has advanced significantly and modern instruments are slimmer and have less bulky ultrasonic transducers at the tip and better video optics. An alternative to dilatation is to use an HFCP. These have been used with some success but are not routinely recommended in this situation because of the lack of penetration and suboptimal nodal imaging. An alternative to dilatation is to use the Olympus MH-908 echoendoscope (Figure 4.12). This conical tipped instrument lacks endoscopic optics and is passed through strictures over a monorail guide wire placed endoscopically. With a diameter of only 7.8 mm, this instrument is capable of traversing all but the tightest senses with no or minimal dilatation.

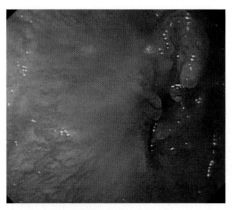

Figure 4.11 Stenosing esophageal carcinoma arising at the esophagogastric junction. Despite dilatation, standard radial EUS echoendoscopes could not traverse the stricture.

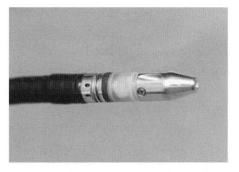

Figure 4.12 Olympus MH-908 esophagoprobe. This 6.9-mm, wire-guided, nonoptical probe can traverse tightest strictures with minimal or no dilatation.

Several studies have demonstrated the equivalent accuracy of this instrument in comparison with standard echoendoscopes with a reported T-staging accuracy of 89% [64,69]. Two series have shown that the use of this instrument permits complete staging (by morphology) in 95% of cases without the need for dilation [70,71].

Another factor limiting EUS performance is its operator dependency [72,73,74,75]. Several studies have demonstrated that endosonographers who have performed more than 50–75 EUS esophageal cancer examinations have good agreement and high accuracy for N staging of esophageal cancer [72,73,74]. The number of procedures performed in a unit is also important. van Vliet *et al.* compared the results in a low-volume center for EUS (each individual endoscopist performed less than 50 EUS staging procedures per year) with those reported from high-volume US EUS centers and found that the sensitivity and specificity for T1 or T2 were lower (58 versus 75–90% and 87 versus 94–97%, respectively) in the low-volume center, while T3 sensitivity was similar (85 versus 88–94%) between the centers, specificity was, however, lower (57 versus 75–90%) [76]. The sensitivity for detecting T4 disease (45 versus 63–89%) and particularly M1a (celiac) lymph nodes (19 versus 72–83%) was particularly poor in the low-volume center.

Future developments

Three-dimensional EUS probes are available, which provide simultaneous dual-plane radial and linear images. This allows measurement of tumor volume and gives excellent views of the relationship of the tumor to surrounding structures. The role of these probes is being investigated and may be of particular use in restaging patients after neoadjuvant therapy.

Bridging the gap between endoscopy and translational research holds great promise for the future. Lymph node samples collected via EUS-FNA have been used to examine epigenetic changes in esophageal cancer [77]. EUS-FNA also allows accurate targeting of tumors. This approach has been used in pilot studies in pancreatic cancer with EUS-guided injection of different antitumor agents directly into the tumor [78,79]; however, to date no studies have been undertaken in esophageal cancer. EUS has also been used to guide radiofrequency ablation in patients with primary, recurrent, or metastatic liver cancer [80], and it may in the future have a role to play in treating metastatic liver lesions from esophageal cancer. EUS can also assist EMR or submucosal dissection techniques by allowing precise placement of the injection needle into the appropriate layer of the esophagus and also ensuring complete separation of the lesion from normal tissue [81,82,83].

The exact role of EUS relative to FDG-PET also needs to be delineated. FDG-PET can be associated with false-positive findings – a situation in which EUS-FNA may be useful. Cost-effectiveness will also need to be examined. At present CT combined with EUS-FNA has been shown to the best cost minimization strategy and may offer more quality-adjusted life years, on average, than any other strategy. PET plus EUS-FNA may be marginally more effective, but also more expensive [62].

Conclusion

EUS, in combination with CT and PET, plays a key role in esophageal cancer staging, particularly in detecting T1 m and T4 disease. Confirmation of N1 status by FNA and detection of M1a disease not detectable by other imaging modalities are other crucial roles for this technique. Optimum staging, however, requires close collaboration and teamwork between specialist radiologists and endoscopists.

REFERENCES

1. American Joint Committee on Cancer. *AJCC Cancer Staging Manual*. (Philadelphia, PA: Lippincott-Raven, 2001), 91–8.
2. V. Vilgrain, D. Mompoint, L. Palazzo, *et al*. Staging of oesophageal carcinoma: comparison of results with endoscopic sonography and CT. *AJR Am J Roentgenol*, **155** (1990), 277–81.
3. T. Rosch. Endosonographic staging of esophageal cancer: a review of literature results. *Gastrointest Endosc Clin N Am*, **5** (1995), 537–47.
4. J. Botet, C. J. Lightdale, G. Zauber, *et al*. Preoperative staging of esophageal cancer: comparison of endoscopic US and dynamic CT. *Radiology*, **181** (1991), 419–25.
5. C. Lightdale and K. G. Kulkarni. Role of endoscopic ultrasonography in the staging and follow-up of esophageal cancer. *J Clin Oncol*, **20** (2005), 4483–9.
6. E. Vazquez-Sequeiros, I. D. Norton, J. E. Clain, *et al*. Impact of endoscopic ultrasound guided fine-needle aspiration on lymph node staging in patients with esophageal carcinoma. *Gastrointest Endosc*, **53** (2001), 751–7.

7. A. Holscher, E. Bollschweiler, P. M. Schneider, *et al.* Early adenocarcinoma in Barrett's oesophagus. *Br J Surg*, **84** (1997), 1470–3.

8. A. Berger and W. J. Scott. Noninvasive staging of esophageal carcinoma. *J Surg Res*, **117** (2004), 127–33.

9. G. Falk, M. F. Catalano, M. V. Sivak, Jr., *et al.*, Endosonography in the evaluation of patients with Barrett's esophagus and high-grade dysplasia. *Gastrointest Endosc*, **40** (1994), 207–12.

10. M. Canto. Barrett's esophagus. *Gastrointest Endosc Clin N Am*, **15** (2005), 83–92.

11. N. Hasegawa, Y. Niwa, T. Arisawa, *et al.* Preoperative staging of superficial esophageal carcinoma: comparison of an ultrasound probe and standard endoscopic ultrasonography. *Gastrointest Endosc*, **44** (1996), 388–93.

12. J. Menzel, N. Hoepffner, H. Nottberg, *et al.* Preoperative staging of esophageal carcinoma: miniprobe sonography versus conventional endoscopic ultrasound in a prospective histopathologically verified study. *Endoscopy*, **31** (1999), 291–7.

13. E. Vazquez-Sequeiros and M. J. Wiersema. High-frequency US catheter-based staging of early esophageal tumors. *Gastrointest Endosc*, **55** (2002), 95–9.

14. M. Fukuda, K. Hirata, H. Natori, *et al.* Endoscopic ultrasonography of the esophagus. *World J Surg*, **24** (2000), 216–26.

15. M. Hunerbein, B. M. Ghadimi, W. Haensch, *et al.* Transendoscopic ultrasound of esophageal and gastric cancer using miniaturized ultrasound catheter probes. *Gastrointest Endosc*, **48** (1998), 371–5.

16. Y. Murata, S. Suzuki, M. Ohta, *et al.* Endoscopic ultrasonography in diagnosis of esophageal carcinoma. *Surg Endosc*, **1** (1996), 11–16.

17. T. Kawano, M. Ohshima, and T. Iwai. Early esophageal carcinoma: endosopic ultrasonography using the Sonoprobe. *Abdom Imaging*, **28** (2003), 477–85.

18. L. Nesje, K. Svanes, A. Viste, *et al.* Comparison of a linear miniature ultrasound probe and a radial scanning echoendoscope in TN staging of esophageal cancer. *Scand J Gastroenterol*, **35** (2000), 997–1002.

19. H. Yanai, T. Yoshida, T. Harada, *et al.* Endoscopic ultrasonography of superficial esophageal cancers using a thin ultrasound probe system equipped with switchable radial and linear scanning modes. *Gastrointest Endosc*, **44** (1996), 578–82.

20. M. Wallace, B. J. Hoffman, A. S. Sahai, *et al.* Imaging of esophageal tumors with a water-filled condom and a catheter US probe. *Gastrointest Endosc*, **51** (2000), 597–600.

21. J. Menzel and W. Domschke. Gastrointestinal miniprobe sonography: the current status. *Am J Gastroenterol*, **95** (2000), 605–16.

22. A. Newnham, M. J. Quinn, P. Babb, *et al.* Trends in oesophageal and gastric cancer incidence, mortality and survival in England and Wales 1971–1998/1999. *Aliment Pharmacol Ther*, **17** (2003), 655–64.

23. P. Pfau, G. G. Ginsberg, R. J. Lew, *et al*. EUS predictors of long-term survival in esophageal carcinoma. *Gastrointest Endosc*, **53** (2001), 463–9.

24. N. Rizk, E. Venkatraman, B. Park, *et al*. The prognostic importance of the number of involved lymph nodes in esophageal cancer: Implications for revisions of the American Joint Committee on Cancer staging system. *J. Thorac. Cardiovasc. Surg*, **132** (2006), 1374–81.

25. J. Roder, R. Busch, H. J. Stein, *et al*. Ratio of invaded to removed lymph nodes as a predictor of survival in squamous cell carcinoma of the esophagus. *Br J Surg*, **81** (1994), 410–13.

26. S. Natsugoe, H. Yoshinaka, M. Shimada, *et al*. Number of lymph node metastases determined by presurgical ultrasound and endoscopic ultrasound is related to prognosis in patients with esophageal carcinoma. *Ann Surg*, **234** (2001), 613–18.

27. W. Killinger, T. W. Rice, D. J. Adelstein, *et al*. Stage II esophageal carcinoma: the significance of T and N. *J Thorac Cardiovasc Surg*, **111** (1996), 935–40.

28. M. Catalano, M. V. Sivak, Jr., T. Rice, *et al*. Endosonographic features predictive of lymph node metastases. *Gastrointest Endosc*, **40** (1994), 442–6.

29. M. Bhutani, R. H. Hawes, and B. J. Hoffman. A comparison of the accuracy of echo features during endoscopic ultrasound (EUS) and EUS-guided fine-needle aspiration for diagnosis of malignant lymph node invasion. *Gastrointest Endosc*, **45** (1997), 474–9.

30. S. Kelly, K. M. Harris, E. Berry, *et al*. A systematic review of the staging performance of endoscopic ultrasound in gastro-oesophageal carcinoma. *Gut*, **49** (2001), 534–9.

31. E. Vazquez-Sequeiros, M. J. Wiersema, J. E. Clain, *et al*. Impact of lymph node staging on therapy of esophageal carcinoma. *Gastoenterology*, **125** (2003), 1626–35.

32. T. Tio, P. Cohen, P. P. Coene, *et al*. Endosonography and computed tomography of oesophageal carcinoma: preoperative classification compared to the new 1987 TNM system. *Gastoenterology*, **96** (1989), 1478–86.

33. T. Rice, G. A. Boyce, and J. M. V. Sivak, Jr. Esophageal ultrasound and the preoperative staging of carcinoma of the esophagus. *J Thorac Cardiovasc Surg*, **101** (1991), 536–43.

34. H. Dittler and J. R. Siewert. Role of endoscopic ultrasonography in esophageal carcinoma. *Endoscopy*, **25** (1993), 156–61.

35. P. Flamen, A. Lerut, E. Van Cutsem, *et al*. Utility of positron emission tomography for the staging of patients with potentially operable esophageal carcinoma. *J Clin Oncol*, **18** (2000), 3203–10.

36. J. Choi, K. H. Lee, Y. M. Shim, *et al*. Improved detection of individual nodal involvement in squamous cell carcinoma of the esophagus by FDG PET. *J Nucl Med*, **41** (2000), 808–15.

37. J. Rasanen, F. I. Sihvo, M. J. Knuuti, *et al*. Prospective analysis of accuracy of PET, CT and EUS in staging of adenocarcinoma of the esophagus and gastroesophageal cancer. *Ann Surg Oncol*, **10** (2003), 954–60.

38. E. Vazquez-Sequeiros, M. J. Levy, J. E. Clain, *et al.* Routine vs. selective EUS-guided FNA approach for preoperative nodal staging of esophageal carcinoma. *Gastrointest Endosc*, **63** (2006), 204–11.

39. C. Reed, G. Mischra, A. V. Sahai, *et al.* Esophageal cancer staging: improved accuracy by endoscopic ultrasound in coeliac lymph nodes. *Ann Thorac Surg*, **67** (1999), 319–22.

40. M. Eloubeidi, M. B. Wallace, C. E. Reed, *et al.* The utility of EUS and EUS-guided fine needle aspiration in detecting coeliac lymph node metastasis in patients with esophageal cancer: a single-center experience. *Gastrointest Endosc*, **54** (2001), 714–19.

41. M. Giovannini, J. F. Seitz, G. Monges, *et al.* Fine-needle aspiration cytology guided by endoscopic ultrasonography: results in 141 patients. *Endoscopy*, **27** (1995), 171–7.

42. D. Williams, A. V. Sahai, L. Aabakken, *et al.* Endoscopic ultrasound guided fine needle aspiration biopsy: a large single centre experience. *Gut*, **44** (1999), 720–6.

43. J. Romagnuolo, J. Scott, R. H. Hawes, *et al.* Helical CT versus EUS with fine needle aspiration for coeliac nodal assessment in patients with esophageal cancer. *Gastrointest Endosc*, **55** (2002), 648–54.

44. K. McGrath, D. Brody, J. Luketich, *et al.* Detection of unsuspected left hepatic lobe metastases during EUS staging of cancer of the esophagus and cardia. *Am J Gastroenterol*, **101** (2006), 1742–6.

45. P. Prasad, N. Schmulewitz, A. Patel, *et al.* Detection of occult liver metastases during EUS for staging of malignancies. *Gastrointest Endosc*, **59** (2004), 49–53.

46. P. Nguyen, J. C. Feng, K. J. Chang. Endoscopic ultrasound (EUS) and EUS-guided fine-needle aspiration (FNA) of liver lesions. *Gastrointest Endosc*, **50** (1999), 357–61.

47. R. Cerfolio, A. S. Bryant, B. Ohja, *et al.* The accuracy of endoscopic ultrasonography with fine-needle aspiration, integrated positron emission tomography with computed tomography, and computed tomography in restaging patients with esophageal cancer after neoadjuvant chemoradiotherapy. *J Thorac Cardiovasc Surg*, **129** (2005), 1232–41.

48. I. Kalha, M. Kaw, N. Fukami, *et al.* The accuracy of endoscopic ultrasound for restaging esophageal carcinoma after chemoradiation therapy. *Cancer*, **101** (2004), 940–7.

49. G. Zuccaro, T. W. Rice, J. Goldblum, *et al.* Endoscopic ultrasound cannot determine suitability for esophagectomy after aggressive chemoradiotherapy for esophageal cancer. *Am J Gastroenterol*, **94** (1999), 906–12.

50. B. Beseth, R. Bedford, W. H. Isacoff, *et al.* Endoscopic ultrasound does not accurately assess pathologic stage of esophageal cancer after neoadjuvant chemoradiotherapy. *Am Surg*, **66** (2000), 827–31.

51. D. Bowrey, G. W. Clark, S. A. Roberts, *et al.* Serial endoscopic ultrasound in the assessment of response to chemoradiotherapy for carcinoma of the esophagus. *J Gastrointest Surg*, **3** (1999), 462–7.

52. N. Hirata, K. Kawamoto, T. Ueyama, *et al.* Using endosonography to assess the effects of neoadjuvant therapy in patients with advanced esophageal cancer. *AJR Am J Roentgenol*, **169** (1997), 485–91. Erratum in: *AJR Am J Roentgenol* 170 (1998), 510.

53. G. Isenberg, A. Chak, M. I. Canto, *et al.* Endoscopic ultrasound in restaging of esophageal cancer after neoadjuvant chemoradiation. *Gastrointest Endosc*, **48** (1998), 158–63.

54. J. Willis, G. S. Cooper, G. Isenberg, *et al.* Correlation of EUS measurement with pathologic assessment of neoadjuvant therapy response in esophageal carcinoma. *Gastrointest Endosc*, **55** (2002), 655–61.

55. A. Chak, M. I. Canto, G. S. Cooper, *et al.* Endosonographic assessment of multimodality therapy predicts survival of esophageal carcinoma patients. *Cancer*, **88** (2000), 1788–95.

56. M. Westerterp, H. L. van Westreenen, J. B. Reitsma, *et al.* Esophageal cancer: CT, endoscopic US and FDG-PET for assessment of response to neoadjuvant therapy: systematic review. *Radiology*, **23** (2005), 841–51.

57. G. Harewood and K. S. Kumar. Assessment of clinical impact of endoscopic ultrasound on esophageal cancer. *J Gastroenterol Hepatol*, **19** (2004), 433–9.

58. S. Preston, G. W. Clark, I. G. Martin, *et al.* Effect of endoscopic ultrasonography on the management of 100 consecutive patients with oesophageal and junctional carcinoma. *Br J Surg*, **90** (2003), 1220–4.

59. A. Ainsworth, M. B. Mortensen, J. Durup, *et al.* Clinical impact of endoscopic ultrasonography at a country hospital. *Endoscopy*, **34** (2002), 447–50.

60. M. Nickl, M. S. Bhutani, M. Catalano, *et al.* Clinical implications of endoscopic ultrasound: the American Endosonography Club Study. *Gastrointest Endosc*, **44** (1996), 371–7.

61. G. C. Harewood and M. J. Wiersema. A cost analysis of endoscopic ultrasound in the evaluation of esophageal cancer. *Am J Gastroenterol*, **97** (2002), 452–8.

62. M. Wallace, P. J. Netter, C. Earle, *et al.* An analysis of multiple staging management strategies for carcinoma of the esophagus: computed tomography, endoscopic ultrasound, positron emission tomography, and thoracoscopy/laparoscopy. *Ann Thorac Surg*, **74** (2002), 1026–32.

63. J. Van Dam, T. W. Rice, M. F. Catalano, *et al.* High grade malignant stricture is predictive of tumor stage. Risks of endosonographic evaluation. *Cancer*, **71** (1993), 2910–17.

64. S. Mallery and J. Van Dam. Increased rate of complete EUS staging of patients with esophageal cancer using the nonoptical, wire-guided echoendoscope. *Gastrointest Endosc*, **50** (1999), 53–7.

65. P. Pfau, G. G. Ginsberg, R. J. Lew, *et al.* Esophageal dilation for endosonographic evaluation of malignant esophageal strictures is safe and effective. *Am J Gastroenterol*, **95** (2000), 2813–15.

66. M. Catalano, J. Van Dam, M. V. Sivak, Jr., *et al.* Malignant esophageal strictures: staging accuracy of endoscopic ultrasonography. *Gastrointest Endosc*, **41** (1995), 535–9.

67. M. Wallace, R. H. Hawes, A. V. Sahai, *et al.* Dilation of malignant esophageal stenosis to allow EUS guided fine-needle aspiration: safety and effect on patient management. *Gastrointest Endosc*, **51** (2000), 309–13.

68. G. Kallimanis, P. K. Gupta, F. H. Al-Kawas, *et al.* Endoscopic ultrasound for staging esophageal cancer, with or without dilation, is clinically important and safe. *Gastrointest Endosc*, **41** (1995), 540–6.

69. K. Binmoeller, H. Seifert, U. Seitz, *et al.* Ultrasonic esophagoprobe for TNM staging of highly stenosing esophageal carcinoma. *Gastrointest Endosc*, **41** (1995), 547–52.

70. V. Dhir, K. M. Mohandas, S. Mehta, *et al.* Endoscopic ultrasound staging of stenotic esophageal cancer: miniprobe, dilation, MH908 or helical computed tomography (CT)? *Gastrointest Endosc*, **56** (2002), S108.

71. C. Vu, L. A. Doig, S. Anderson, *et al.* Large series Western European experience with the Olympus MH908 slim-probe shows greater complete staging of esophageal cancer without the need for dilatation (abstract). *Gastrointest Endosc*, **59** (2004), AB213.

72. M. Catalano, M. V. Sivak, Jr., R. A. Bedford, *et al.* Observer variation and reproducibility for endoscopic ultrasonography. *Gastrointest Endosc*, **41** (1995), 115–20.

73. L. Palazzo and P. Burtin. Interobserver variation in tumor staging. *Gastrointest Endosc Clin N Am*, **5** (1995), 559–67.

74. P. Fockens, J. H. van den Brande, H. M. van Dullemen, *et al.* Endosonographic T-staging of esophageal carcinoma: a learning curve. *Gastrointest Endosc*, **44** (1996), 58–62.

75. T. Schlick, A. Heintz, and T. Junginger. The examiner's learning effect and its influence on the quality of endoscopic ultrasonography in carcinomas of the esophagus and gastric cardia. *Surg Endosc*, **13** (1999), 894–8.

76. E. P. M. van Vliet, M. J. C. Eijkemans, J.-W. Poley, *et al.* Staging of esophageal carcinoma in a low-volume EUS center compared with reported results from high-volume centers. *Gastrointest Endosc*, **63** (2006), 938–47.

77. M. Pellise, A. Castells, A. Gines, *et al.* Detection of lymph node micrometastases by gene promoter hypermethylation in samples obtained by endosonography-guided fine-needle aspiration biopsy. *Clin Cancer Res*, **10** (2004), 4444–9.

78. K. Chang, P. T. Nguyen, J. A. Thompson, *et al.* Phase 1 clinical trial of allogeneic mixed lymphocyte culture (cytoimplant) delivered by endoscopic ultrasound-guided fine needle-injection in patients with advanced pancreatic carcinoma. *Cancer*, **88** (2000), 1325–35.

79. J. Hecht, R. Bedford, J. L. Abbruzzese, *et al.* A phase I/II trial of intramural endoscopic ultrasound injection of ONYX-015 with intravenous gemcitabine in unresectable pancreatic carcinoma. *Clin Cancer Res*, **9** (2003), 555–61.

80. S. Goldberg, S. Mallery, G. S. Gazelle, *et al.* EUS-guided radiofrequency ablation in the pancreas: results in a porcine model. *Gastrointest Endosc*, **50** (1999), 392–401.

81. S. Sun and M. Wang. Use of endoscopic ultrasound-guided injection in endoscopic resection of submucosal tumors. *Endoscopy*, **34** (2002), 82–5.

82. A. Fritscher-Ravens, N. Appleyard, and P. Swain. Real time echoendoscopic control of submucosal resection and polypectomy (abstract). *Gastrointest Endosc*, **55** (2002), AB254.

83. A. Fritscher-Ravens, A. Moss, D. Mukherjee, *et al*. Real time (miniprobe) EUS controlled endoscopic submucosal resection (abstract). *Gastrointest Endosc*, **53** (2001), AB128.

5

CT in Esophageal Cancer

Naama R. Bogot and Leslie Eisenbud Quint

Introduction

Cross-sectional imaging with computer tomography (CT) and magnetic resonance imaging (MRI) has no significant role in diagnosing esophageal cancer, although it is complementary to endoscopy, barium studies, endoscopic ultrasound (EUS), and positron emission tomography (PET) imaging in the staging of esophageal cancer. Accurate staging is necessary in order to prompt appropriate curative or palliative therapy. While CT and MRI are insensitive for delineating tumor invasion into and through the esophageal wall, these modalities play a role in estimating the esophageal tumor bulk, evaluating for local spread into adjacent structures, and diagnosing distant metastases, when present. Cross-sectional imaging also has an important role in the follow-up of esophageal cancer patients after treatment, to assess response to chemoradiotherapy and to evaluate recurrence after treatment [1].

Anatomy and staging

Knowledge of esophageal anatomy is important both for understanding how esophageal cancer spreads and for staging purposes. The esophageal wall consists of four layers: mucosa, submucosa, muscularis propria, and adventitia (Figure 5.1). There is no serosa to serve as a barrier between the esophagus and the surrounding structures; lack of a serosa facilitates tumor spread through the esophageal wall into adjacent structures. A rich plexus of lymphatics encircles the entire length of the esophagus, enabling lymphatic spread of tumor to mediastinal, cervical, and upper abdominal lymph nodes (Figure 5.2). An experimental study showed that dye injected into the esophageal wall at one level may drain to lymph nodes at all other levels of the esophagus in some patients and also frequently drains directly

Carcinoma of the Esophagus, ed. Sheila C. Rankin. Published by Cambridge University Press. © Cambridge University Press 2008.

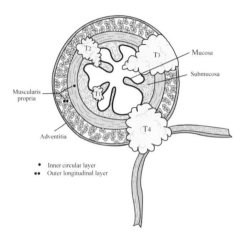

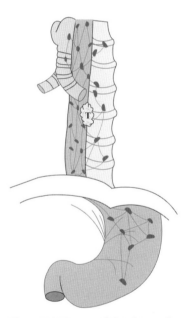

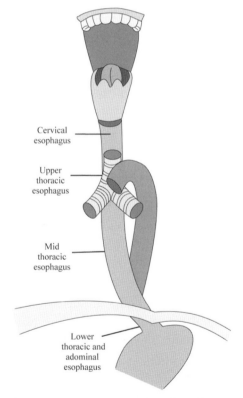

Figure 5.1 Diagram showing the four layers of the esophageal wall: mucosa, submucosa, muscularis propria, and adventitia, as well as extraesophageal fat. T1 tumors extend no deeper than the submucosa. T2 tumors invade the muscularis propria. T3 tumors invade into or through the adventitia. T4 lesions invade adjacent structures.

Figure 5.2 Diagram of the plexus of lymphatics that encircles the entire length of the esophagus, enabling lymphatic spread of tumor to mediastinal, cervical, and upper abdominal lymph nodes. T, tumor.

Figure 5.3 The esophagus is divided into four anatomic regions for reporting and staging purposes: cervical, and upper, mid, and lower thoracic portions.

into the thoracic duct, potentially leading to hematogenous metastases [2]. Because of these features, "skip metastases" are not uncommon, meaning that distant sites may be involved without involvement of lymph nodes close to the primary tumor. In addition, advanced disease is frequently seen at initial clinical presentation [3]. Only about 24% of esophagus cancer cases are diagnosed while the cancer is still confined to the primary site (localized stage); 29% are diagnosed after the cancer has spread to regional lymph nodes or directly beyond the primary site; 30% are diagnosed after the cancer has already metastasized (distant stage); and for the remaining 17% the staging information is unknown [4].

The esophagus is divided into four anatomic regions for reporting and staging purposes (Figure 5.3). The cervical portion extends from the cricoid cartilage to the thoracic inlet. The thoracic esophagus extends from the thoracic inlet to the gastroesophageal junction and is divided into three regions: upper, mid, and lower. The upper thoracic esophagus extends from the thoracic inlet to the carina; the mid thoracic esophagus from the carina to the diaphragm; and the lower thoracic and abdominal esophagus (which measures approximately 3 cm in length) from the diaphragm down to and including the gastroesophageal junction [5,6]. The cervical esophagus ends approximately 18 cm from the incisors; the upper, mid, and lower thoracic esophagus end at approximately 24, 32, and 40 cm from the incisors, respectively.

Staging Classification

The International Union Against Cancer (UICC) and American Joint Committee on Cancer (AJCC) have staged esophageal cancer using the TNM system whereby T categorizes the depth of invasion into or through the esophageal wall (Figure 5.1), N the status of regional lymph nodes, and M metastases to distant sites (Table 5.1) [5]. Stage groupings of the TNM system, based on prognosis, are listed in Table 5.2 [5].

Regional lymph nodes are determined according to the level of the primary esophageal tumor according to the National Comprehensive Cancer Network (NCCN) Clinical Practice Guidelines [7]. For example, regional sites for cervical esophageal primaries include the cervical, scalene, supraclavicular, and mediastinal lymph nodes. The regional sites for upper and middle intrathoracic esophageal tumors are mediastinal, hilar, and left gastric lymph nodes, and for lower thoracic and abdominal tumors are mediastinal, left gastric, common hepatic, diaphragmatic, and splenic nodes. Lymph node metastases to any other sites constitute distant metastatic (M1) disease.

Table 5.1   TNM staging of esophageal cancer

Primary tumor (T)	
T0	No evidence of primary tumor
Tis	Carcinoma *in situ*
T1	Tumor confined to mucosa or invades lamina propria or submucosa
T2	Tumor invades muscularis propria
T3	Tumor invades adventitia
T4	Tumor invades adjacent structures
Regional lymph nodes (N)	
N0	No regional lymph node metastasis
N1	Regional lymph node metastasis
Distant metastasis (M)	
M0	No distant metastasis
M1	Distant metastasis

Table 5.2   Esophageal cancer stage grouping

Stage grouping	T	N	M
Stage 0	Tis	N0	M0
Stage I	T1	N0	M0
Stage IIA	T2	N0	M0
	T3	N0	M0
Stage IIB	T1	N1	M0
	T2	N1	M0
Stage III	T3	N1	M0
	T4	Any N	M0
Stage IV	Any T	Any N	M1
Stage IVA	Any T	Any N	M1a
Stage IVB	Any T	Any N	M1b

Only for upper thoracic and for lower thoracic primary tumors, M1 is broken down into M1a and M1b categories (cervical and mid thoracic primary tumors have no such breakdown) (Table 5.3). Tumor spread to cervical lymph nodes from an upper thoracic primary neoplasm falls into the M1a category; spread to any other nonregional lymph nodes represents M1b disease. Similarly, celiac axis lymph node metastases confer M1a status upon primary tumors located in the

Table 5.3   M1 disease according to primary tumor level

Tumors of the upper thoracic esophagus	
M1a	Metastasis in cervical nodes
M1b	Other distant metastasis
Tumors of the mid thoracic esophagus	
M1a	Not applicable
M1b	Nonregional lymph nodes and/or other distant metastasis
Tumors of the lower thoracic esophagus	
M1a	Metastasis in celiac lymph nodes
M1b	Other distant metastasis

lower thoracic esophagus, whereas spread to any other nonregional lymph nodes represents M1b disease. Patients with M1a disease have a better prognosis than those with M1b disease and are therefore generally felt to represent surgical candidates. However, in patients with adenocarcinoma of the lower esophagus this distinction has been debated [8]. Although patients with M1a disease had a statistically significantly improved prognosis in one study, it was of limited clinical significance, as the median survival for M1a stage disease was 11 months, compared to 5 months for M1b disease.

Patients with newly diagnosed esophageal cancer often present with distant metastases. In a series by Quint *et al.*, 18% of patients presented with M1 disease. Distant metastases were most commonly diagnosed in upper abdominal lymph nodes (45%), followed by liver (35%) and lung (20%). Less commonly, distant metastases were seen in cervical/supraclavicular lymph nodes, bone, adrenal glands, peritoneum, brain, pericardium, pleura, stomach, pancreas, spleen, soft tissues, and kidney [9].

Computed tomography

Diagnosis of esophageal cancer

Esophageal cancers usually manifest as focal wall thickening at CT, either concentric or eccentric [10]. The normal wall width of the distended esophagus is approximately 3 mm (Figure 5.4); a width of 5 mm or greater is considered abnormal [11,12] (Figure 5.5). In order to obtain better delineation of the thickness of the esophageal wall at CT, the esophagus may be opacified with a dilute

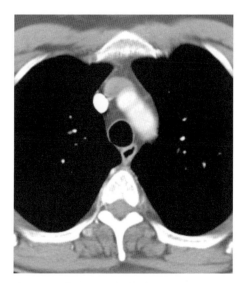

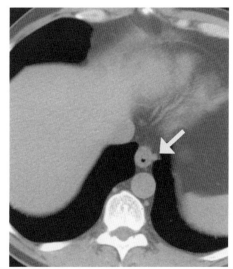

Figure 5.4 CT shows a distended normal esophagus with wall width less than 5 mm.

Figure 5.5 In a 46-year-old man with distal esophageal adenocarcinoma, CT shows distal esophageal thickening, representing the primary tumor, as well as a prominent paraesophageal lymph node (arrow), suggestive of regional nodal metastatic disease.

barium paste and/or distended by ingestion of effervescent granules, immediately before scanning. However, CT is not generally used for the primary diagnosis of esophageal cancer, because wall thickening is a nonspecific finding and may be related to benign conditions such esophagitis due to radiation therapy, infection, or reflux [13]. Furthermore, small cancers may not even be visible on CT, particularly if the esophagus is collapsed [14]. Recent preliminary work, however, using triple-phase dynamic CT, has suggested that tumor may be visible without wall thickening and is best seen during the late arterial phase of the contrast injection [15] (Figure 5.6).

Evaluation of tumor size

Tumor bulk may have prognostic implications. It was shown by Lefor *et al.* that when the tumor is greater than 3 cm in width, there is a higher likelihood of extraesophageal spread, including mediastinal invasion and spread to abdominal lymph nodes and liver [16]. There is a tendency to overestimate tumor length on axial images provided by CT. In an older CT study, Quint and colleagues

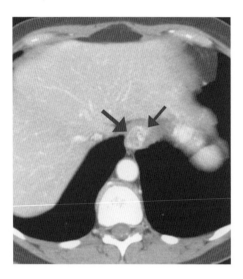

Figure 5.6 In a 66-year-old woman with esophageal adenocarcinoma, CT shows an enhancing distal esophageal mass (arrows).

compared tumor lengths on CT to lengths on the resected surgical specimens and found overestimations ranging between 1.5 – and 7.5 cm in nearly 50% of patients [17]. In addition to assessing the esophageal tumor length, in some patients it is important to assess the degree of tumor extension into the stomach: if a large part of the stomach is involved, then it is not suitable for use as a gastric conduit. In this situation, the surgeons need to be aware that a colon interposition may be necessary, and the patient needs colonic cleansing in preparation for surgery. Unfortunately, CT is not generally reliable in evaluating for gastric tumor extension. These problems may be overcome in the future with better esophageal and gastric distention techniques and newer generation CT scanners, using thin sections with high-resolution volumetric data, yielding detailed multiplanar and 3D reconstructions and virtual endoscopy images [14,18].

Primary tumor (T) staging

Unlike EUS, CT is incapable of distinguishing the layers of the esophageal wall in order to determine the depth of tumor invasion, i.e., T1 versus T2 disease (Figure 5.7). Gross tumor invasion into mediastinal fat may be diagnosed at CT (T3 disease), manifesting as abnormal soft tissue in the mediastinal fat, with or without obliteration of fat planes between the esophagus and adjacent mediastinal structures [10,19] (Figure 5.8). However, most investigators believe that CT is unreliable in detecting or excluding minimal fat invasion [10,19] (Figure 5.9).

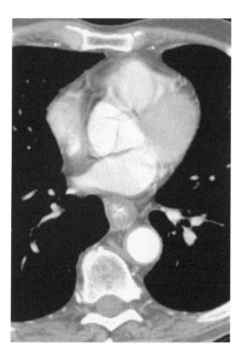

Figure 5.7 In a 63-year-old man with esophageal adenocarcinoma, stage T2 according to endoscopic ultrasonography, CT shows circumferential esophageal wall thickening, without delineation of the layers of the esophageal wall.

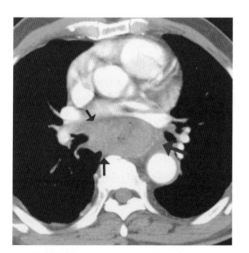

Figure 5.8 In a 74-year-old man with esophageal squamous cell carcinoma, CT shows a mid esophageal mass with soft tissue extending into the surrounding mediastinum (arrows), consistent with gross T3 disease.

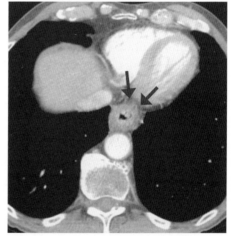

Figure 5.9 In a 70-year-old man with esophageal adenocarcinoma, CT shows circumferential thickening of the esophageal wall with soft tissue stranding extending into the surrounding mediastinal fat (arrows), suggesting T3 disease. This was confirmed by pathological evaluation of the esophagectomy specimen.

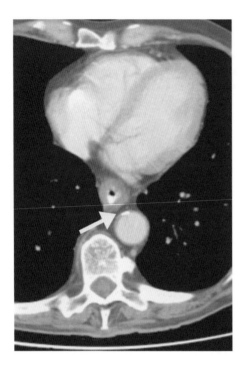

Figure 5.10 In a 63-year-old man with esophageal adenocarcinoma, fat plane between the esophageal cancer and the aorta (arrow) indicates lack of aortic invasion.

On the other hand, one recent study found that distention of the esophagus with effervescent granules and postprocessing the data with multiplanar reconstructions did lead to accurate assessment of extraesophageal tumor spread [14]. In general, the major role of CT is to detect local tumor invasion into adjacent structures (T4 disease) and/or presence of distant metastases (M1), suggesting inoperability. The presence of a fat plane between an esophageal tumor and an adjacent mediastinal structure (e.g., central airway, aorta, and pericardium) is an accurate indicator of lack of invasion of the structure (Figure 5.10). However, the converse is not necessarily true: lack of a fat plane is not diagnostic for invasion (T4 disease) in either cachectic patients or those with normal body weight. Moreover, adjacent fat planes are sometimes obscured in patients who have undergone radiation therapy.

Deep invasion of the aortic wall is unresectable, whereas invasion limited to the adventitia is generally resectable [20]. Various CT techniques and criteria have been suggested to help diagnose or exclude unresectable aortic invasion. For example, prone positioning has been advocated as a way to separate the tumor from the aorta, thus allowing exclusion of aortic invasion [21]. An older study reported that contact between the mass and the aorta over more than 90° of the aortic circumference was 80% accurate for diagnosing aortic invasion [22]. A somewhat newer

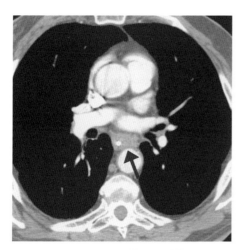

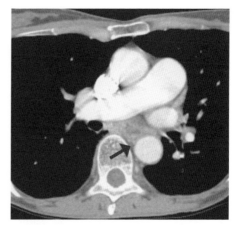

Figure 5.11 In a 73-year-old man with esophageal adenocarcinoma, CT shows a thickened esophagus surrounding a feeding tube. Loss of the fat plane between the cancer and the aorta (arrow) suggests that aortic invasion may be present; no invasion was present at surgery.

Figure 5.12 In a 61-year-old woman with esophageal squamous cell carcinoma, CT demonstrates circumferential thickening of the esophagus, loss of the fat plane between the esophagus and the aorta, and obliteration of the normal fatty triangle between the esophagus, aorta, and spine (arrow), suggesting that aortic invasion may be present; no invasion was present at surgery.

study found that obliteration of the normal fatty triangle located between the spine, esophagus, and aorta showed a sensitivity of 100% and specificity of 82% in this setting [23]. Unfortunately, however, these criteria do not appear to be reliable in clinical practice, and other studies have reported lower accuracies; for example, Lehr *et al.* found sensitivity, specificity, and accuracy figures of 6, 85, and 58%, respectively [24]. Thus, suspected aortic invasion is difficult to prove preoperatively, and in most cases, this determination is a surgical one (Figures 5.11 and 5.12). Fortunately, however, unresectable aortic invasion is a very rare finding.

Unlike aortic invasion, tumor spread into the central airways is not rare and should always be considered in a patient with an upper or mid thoracic primary tumor. Flattening or indentation of the wall of the trachea or left mainstem bronchus by an adjacent esophageal mass (particularly on inspiratory images) is suggestive of invasion, although this finding may be caused by simple mass effect upon the membranous portion of the airway, without invasion [25] (Figure 5.13). Bronchial wall thickening is suggestive of involvement; frank abnormal soft tissue in the lumen of the airway or a fistula between the esophagus and the airway are specific, if extremely uncommon, findings of airway invasion. Overall, the reported

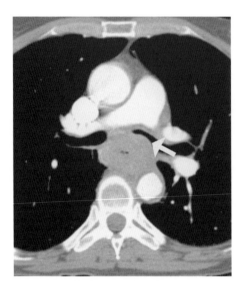

Figure 5.13 In a 57-year-old woman with esophageal adenocarcinoma, CT shows a mid esophageal mass that compresses the left mainstem bronchus (arrow). Bronchial invasion was confirmed bronchoscopically.

sensitivity for tracheobronchial involvement ranges from 31 to 100%, specificity from 68 to 98%, and accuracies range from 74 to 97% [25]. Imaging features suggesting invasion should be further evaluated with bronchoscopy and confirmed with biopsy. Pericardial invasion is suggested by pericardial thickening and/or effusion, obliteration of the fat plane between the tumor and the pericardium, or mass effect upon the pericardium [10,26]. Extensive invasion is unresectable and minimal invasion may be resectable.

Regional lymph node (N) staging

Diagnosing metastatic disease to regional lymph nodes with CT is limited for two major reasons. First, a bulky primary esophageal mass may obscure adjacent, involved lymph nodes [26]. Second diagnosis of lymph node disease is based solely on size criteria. However, enlarged nodes may be benign and reactive in nature, whereas small nodes may harbor microscopic metastases. Several size criteria for lymph node enlargement have been suggested. Traditionally, 10 mm has been considered the upper normal limit for paraesophageal lymph nodes. For subdiaphragmatic nodes, an upper normal threshold of 8 mm has been used, with nodes between 6 and 8 mm considered as indeterminate [27]. However, more recently, Schroder and colleagues have found these figures to be overestimations [28]. In a histopathological study of specimens from 40 patients with esophageal squamous cell carcinoma, 1196 lymph nodes were analyzed, finding 129 lymph nodes with metastatic infiltration.

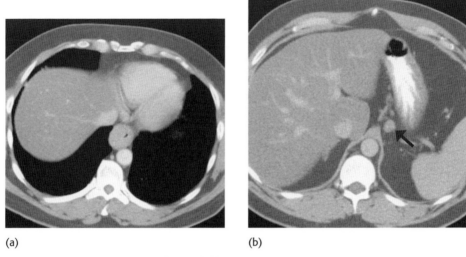

(a)   (b)

Figure 5.14 In a 43-year-old man with newly diagnosed distal esophageal adenocarcinoma, CT shows distal esophageal thickening, representing the primary tumor (a). There was metastatic disease to regional lymph nodes in the gastrohepatic ligament (arrow on (b)).

Average maximum lymph node diameters were 5.1 mm ($\pm$3.8 mm) for tumor-free lymph nodes and 6.7 mm ($\pm$4.2 mm) for tumor-containing lymph nodes. Furthermore, only 9.3% of all resected lymph nodes measured 10 mm or more in maximal diameter. In addition, there was no significant correlation between lymph node size and the frequency of nodal metastases [28].

Recent studies using helical CT have demonstrated varied results in the detection of regional lymph nodes metastases, with sensitivities of 11–69%, specificities of 71.4–95%, and accuracies of 65.6–83% [29,30,31] (Figure 5.14). Criteria for diagnosing lymph node involvement varied among these studies. For example, Wu and colleagues considered lymph nodes as positive if the short axis was greater than 10 mm [29]. Yoon used the same size criteria for all lymph node stations excluding hilar lymph nodes, which were considered enlarged if they measured 10 mm in any axis [30]. On the other hand, Kato and colleagues considered lymph nodes involved if the long axis exceeded 10 mm [31].

Distant metastatic disease (M) staging

Romagnuolo *et al.* compared helical CT to EUS for celiac lymph node evaluation, using aspiration cytology results as proof [32]. In this study, helical CT did poorly, with sensitivity of 53%, specificity of 86%, positive predictive value of 67%, and

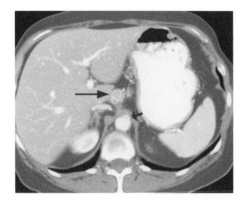

Figure 5.15 In a 66-year-old woman with distal esophageal adenocarcinoma, an enlarged celiac axis lymph node is seen at CT (long arrow). Biopsy confirmed tumor involvement consistent with M1a disease. Origin of celiac axis is indicated by short arrow. (The primary tumor is shown in Figure 5.6.)

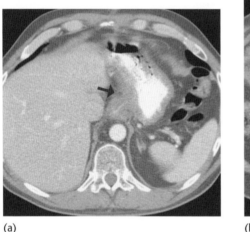

(a)

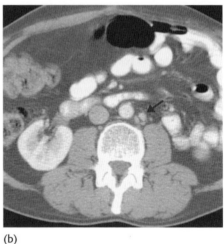

(b)

Figure 5.16 In a 47-year-old man with esophageal adenocarcinoma, CT shows the primary tumor in the distal esophagus and gastroesophageal junction (arrow on (a)). A small left paraaortic lymph (arrow on (b)) was FDG avid at PET scanning (not shown), representing a distant lymph node metastasis consistent with M1b disease.

negative predictive value of 77% (Figure 5.15). Regretfully, the size criterion for lymph node enlargement at CT was not mentioned.

CT scanning is often useful for detection of distant nodal metastatic disease in paraaortic regions and in nonnodal sites (Figures 5.16 and 5.17). The sensitivity for detection of hepatic metastases from gastrointestinal (GI) primary tumors is reported to be approximately 70–80% [33,34]. Interestingly (and surprisingly), a recent meta-analysis showed no significant difference in weighted sensitivity between nonhelical and helical CT [34]. CT scanning of patients with esophageal carcinoma should include a contrast-enhanced CT of the chest and abdomen, with

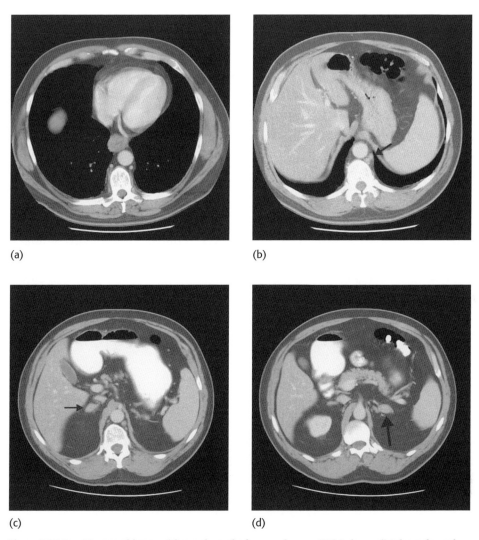

(a)

(b)

(c)

(d)

Figure 5.17 In a 52-year-old man with esophageal adenocarcinoma, CT (a) shows distal esophageal thickening, representing the primary tumor. Metastases were seen in retrocrural lymph nodes (arrow on (b)), right adrenal (arrow on (c)) and left adrenal (arrow on (d)) consistent with M1b disease.

dedicated liver technique to optimize visualization of hepatic metastases. Among 201 CT examinations performed for staging purposes, Gollub and colleagues found that none of the pelvic CT scans affected patient management and concluded that it is therefore unnecessary to perform pelvic CT as part of the staging workup [35].

In spite of CT limitations in showing the local and regional extent of esophageal tumor, multiple studies have demonstrated good correlation between CT staging and patient outcome. Halverson *et al.* evaluated CT examinations from 89 patients and found that CT evidence of mediastinal invasion (specifically tracheal and aortic invasion) or abdominal metastases predicted unfavorable patient outcome [36]. Similarly, Unger *et al.* reported that in patients treated with chemotherapy and radiation therapy, long-term survival correlated indirectly with local extent of the tumor and the presence of distant metastases [37]. Ampil and colleagues found positive correlation between lower CT stage and better prognosis [38].

Magnetic resonance imaging

Several authors have reported that there is no real difference in staging accuracy between MRI and CT for esophageal cancer [23,29,39]. MRI is more costly than CT and less widely available; in addition, it is more difficult to perform, as respiratory and cardiac gating and control of swallowing are needed, in order to optimize images and avoid motion artifacts. Therefore, MRI is rarely used at most institutions for routine staging [26,40].

Workup guidelines

Multiple staging modalities are available for evaluating patients with newly diagnosed esophageal cancer. The following guidelines are followed by multiple authors, yet may be varied according to local preferences and availability of imaging technology [10,41]. Patients should initially undergo a history and physical examination, in order to detect gross evidence of metastatic disease. In addition, complete upper GI endoscopy or barium upper GI series is indicated to assess for mucosal extent of disease. A CT of the chest and abdomen with bolus administration of intravenous contrast should then be performed to evaluate the primary tumor for T4 disease and to look for lymph node, visceral, and other distant metastatic disease. If the CT shows no distant metastases, and if the tumor is in the cervical, upper thoracic, or mid thoracic esophagus, bronchoscopy is generally performed to assess for airway invasion. PET has been shown to be more accurate than CT in diagnosing distant metastases [34]. Therefore, if the disease appears to be resectable at CT, patients may then undergo PET scanning for detection of occult distant metastases; suspicious lesions should be biopsied for confirmation of disease. Assuming the PET study shows no evidence of distant metastatic disease, a patient may then be examined with EUS for better T and N stage evaluation; suspicious lymph nodes detected by EUS (regional or celiac axis) should undergo EUS-guided fine-needle aspiration (EUS-FNA) biopsy.

At some institutions, patients with T1N0 disease on EUS and M0 disease on CT and PET will undergo surgery, whereas those with deeper extent of tumor and/or tumor-involved regional lymph nodes undergo neoadjuvant chemoradiation therapy followed by surgery. M1 disease is usually treated nonsurgically, with chemoradiotherapy. Some centers perform laparoscopy to look for occult abdominal metastases, particularly for tumors arising at the gastroesophageal junction [42,43].

A cost-effectiveness study comparing CT, EUS-FNA, PET, and thoracoscopy/laparoscopy found that CT plus EUS-FNA was the most inexpensive strategy and offered more quality-adjusted life years, on average, than all other strategies except for PET plus EUS-FNA [44]. The latter strategy, although slightly more effective, was also more expensive. The authors recommended the use of PET plus EUS-FNA unless resources are scarce or PET is unavailable [44].

Assessment of Response to Neoadjuvant Therapy

CT has been used to assess response to neoadjuvant chemotherapy and radiation therapy, with mixed results. Using the Miller criteria to assess for response (e.g., partial response means reduction of 50% in tumor load on two examinations obtained 4 weeks apart, with no new lesions) [45], Walker *et al.* compared preoperative CT to resected specimens in order to evaluate response to chemotherapy [46]. These authors found a wide discrepancy between CT and pathological response rates: 48% of patients had complete or partial response on CT, compared to 90% on pathological examination. They concluded that change on CT correctly predicted pathological response, but the lack of response on CT did not preclude pathological regression. In a more recent study using helical CT with gaseous esophageal distention, no correlation was found between postchemotherapy tumor volume reduction at CT and either pathological response or patient survival [47]. However, a study by Beer and colleagues reported that volumetric tumor measurements performed 2 weeks after initiation of neoadjuvant chemotherapy predicted histopathological tumor response with 100% sensitivity and 53% specificity [48]. Thus, results have been mixed, to date, in this setting.

Recurrent esophageal cancer

Frequency and timing of recurrence

The majority of patients with newly diagnosed esophageal cancer already have tumor spread outside of the esophageal wall into adjacent mediastinal tissues or to distant locations [4]. Due to the systemic nature of the disease in most patients, overall 5-year survival is dismal, approximating 13%, and tumor recurrence rates after palliative or attempted curative treatment are extremely high [49]. Not surprisingly, higher T and N stages of the primary tumor correlate with higher recurrence rates [50,51]. More than 50% of patients will recur within the first year after initial therapy, and most patients will die from recurrent tumor [51]. Proven tumor recurrences may be treated with chemotherapy.

Location of recurrence

Recurrent esophageal carcinoma is usually multifocal, both locoregional and distant, regardless of the type of therapy [52,53] (Figures 5.18 and 5.19). After surgery, locoregional recurrences are generally extragastric, in the mediastinum, or in upper abdominal lymph nodes. Occasionally, tumors recur in the intrathoracic stomach or at the esophagogastric anastomosis. There does not appear to be correlation between the craniocaudal level of the primary neoplasm and that of the recurrence, likely because of extensive tumor spread in periesophageal lymphatics before the time of esophagectomy [52]. In addition, distant metastasis can occur without local lymph node metastases, presumably because lymphatic and hematogenous dissemination occur independently [54]. In one series, distant metastases were found without locoregional lymph node spread in

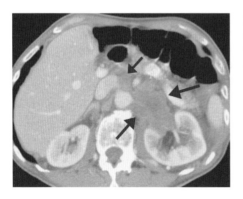

Figure 5.18 In a 77-year-old man with recurrent esophageal adenocarcinoma, CT shows recurrent tumor 4 years after esophagectomy in paraaortic and left renal hilar lymph nodes (arrows).

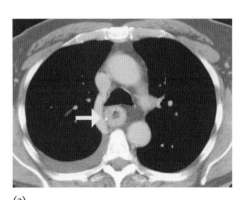
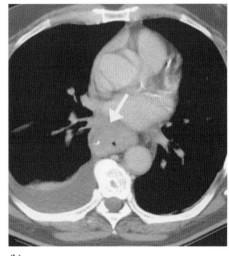

(a)   (b)

Figure 5.19 In a 69-year-old man with recurrent esophageal adenocarcinoma, CT obtained 3 years after esophagectomy shows a normal appearing gastric interposition in the mid thorax (arrow on (a)). However, a more caudal image (b) shows marked thickening of the stomach (arrow); this represented biopsy-proven recurrent tumor.

40% of patients with recurrent disease [51]. According to a CT study, the most common locations for distant recurrences are abdominal lymph nodes, lung, liver, pleura, and adrenal glands, in decreasing order of frequency. Less common locations include cervical lymph nodes, peritoneum, and bone [52]. A recent autopsy study characterizing the frequency and distribution of disease following "curative" esophagectomy detected tumor in 63% of patients [55]. Interestingly, 43% of patients who died of disease not related to esophageal cancer had tumor recurrence. Lymphatic and hematogenous spread was seen in nearly equal proportions (42 and 40% of patients, respectively). Serosal and local recurrences were each found in 26% of patients. Thoracic lymph node spread was more common than abdominal nodal spread, which was, in turn, more common than cervical nodal disease. Thoracic nodal disease was seen most frequently in pulmonary hilar nodes.

Follow-up imaging

The overall accuracy of CT for detection of recurrence is reported to be about 87% [52]. Routine surveillance CT scanning is not generally performed after definitive

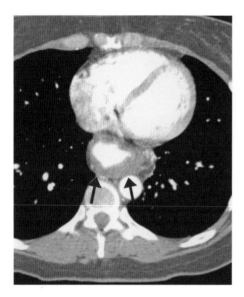

Figure 5.20 In a 44-year-old woman, 2 years after esophagectomy for esophageal adenocarcinoma, CT demonstrates diffuse thickening of the intrathoracic stomach (arrows). Upper endoscopy revealed no abnormality, and the cause of the gastric thickening was unknown.

treatment. Rather, imaging is reserved for those patients with signs and/or symptoms suspicious for recurrent disease.

Benign findings simulating tumor recurrence

Benign CT findings may occasionally simulate recurrent disease (Figure 5.20). For example, focal or diffuse thickening of the intrathoracic stomach may be the result of incomplete distention or posttherapy edema [52,56], and focal mass-like soft tissue at the anastomosis may be due to a benign anastomotic stricture. Mediastinal fat infiltration may represent postoperative changes in the first 3 months after surgery but is not usual thereafter [56]. Isolated pleural and pericardial effusions are often postsurgical or postradiation in nature, rather than neoplastic; however, such effusions should be viewed with suspicion if there is associated soft-tissue thickening and/or nodularity, or if the effusion is a new finding several months or years after therapy, or there is evidence of recurrence elsewhere [52].

One published study compared MRI and CT for diagnosing tumor recurrence following transhiatal esophagectomy in 23 patients. The results demonstrated better sensitivity for CT in detecting lung metastases and better sensitivity for MRI in detecting bone metastases and gastric wall thickening. However, overall there was no significant difference in sensitivity, specificity, or accuracy when evaluating multiple parameters and sites for disease recurrence [57].

Conclusion

Esophageal carcinoma tends to have spread beyond the esophageal wall at the time of diagnosis, either directly to periesophageal tissues, to adjacent or remote lymph nodes, and/or to distant sites. As a result, patients with this disease usually have a dismal prognosis, and only patients with limited disease are suitable for potentially curative surgery. CT has limited value in diagnosing tumor spread across the layers of the esophageal wall. Nevertheless, it has a major role in staging local spread in the mediastinum, as well as metastases to lymph nodes and remote sites, thereby helping to determine which patients are suitable for surgery. CT may be useful for evaluating response to chemotherapy and radiation therapy and for evaluation of tumor recurrence after therapy.

REFERENCES

1. R. B. Iyer, P. M. Silverman, E. P. Tamm, J. S. Dunnington, and R. A. DuBrow. Diagnosis, staging, and follow-up of esophageal cancer. *AJR Am J Roentgenol*, **181** (2003), 785–93.
2. M. Riquet, M. Saab, F. Le Pimpec Barthes, and G. Hidden. Lymphatic drainage of the esophagus in the adult. *Surg Radiol Anat*, **15** (1993), 209–11.
3. A. Sharma, P. Fidias, L. A. Hayman, *et al.* Patterns of lymphadenopathy in thoracic malignancies. *Radiographics*, **24** (2004), 419–34.
4. SEER NCI. Cancer of the Esophagus. http://seer.cancer.gov/statfacts/html/esoph.html (2006).
5. AJCC. *Cancer Staging Handbook.* (New York: Springer, 2002).
6. M. G. Patti, W. Gantert, and L. W. Way. Surgery of the esophagus. Anatomy and physiology. *Surg Clin North Am*, **77** (1997), 959–70.
7. NCCN Clinical Practice Guidelines in Oncology. www.nccn.org (2005).
8. N. A. Christie, T. W. Rice, M. M. DeCamp, *et al.* M1a/M1b esophageal carcinoma: clinical relevance. *J Thorac Cardiovasc Surg*, **118** (1999), 900–7.
9. L. E. Quint, L. M. Hepburn, I. R. Francis, R. I. Whyte, and M. B. Orringer. Incidence and distribution of distant metastases from newly diagnosed esophageal carcinoma. *Cancer*, **76** (1995), 1120–5.
10. T. W. Rice. Clinical staging of esophageal carcinoma. CT, EUS, and PET. *Chest Surg Clin N Am*, **10** (2000), 471–85.

11. H. van Overhagen and C. D. Becker. Diagnosis and staging of carcinoma of the esophagus and gastroesophageal junction, and detection of postoperative recurrence, by computed tomography. In *Neoplasms of the Digestive Tract. Imaging, Staging and Management*, ed. M. A. Meyers. (Philadelphia, PA: Lippincott-Raven, 1998), 31–48.

12. M. D. Halber and R. H. Daffner. Thompson W M. CT of the esophagus: I. Normal appearance. *AJR Am J Roentgenol*, **133** (1979), 1047–50.

13. J. W. Reinig, J. H. Stanley, and S. I. Schabel. CT evaluation of thickened esophageal walls. *AJR Am J Roentgenol*, **140** (1983), 931–4.

14. V. Panebianco, H. Grazhdani, F. Iafrate, *et al*. 3D CT protocol in the assessment of the esophageal neoplastic lesions: can it improve TNM staging? *Eur Radiol*, **16** (2006), 414–21.

15. S. Umeoka, T. Koyama, K. Togashi, *et al*. Esophageal cancer: evaluation with triple-phase dynamic CT – initial experience. *Radiology*, **239** (2006), 777–83.

16. A. T. Lefor, M. M. Merino, S. M. Steinberg, *et al*. Computerized tomographic prediction of extraluminal spread and prognostic implications of lesion width in esophageal carcinoma. *Cancer*, **62** (1988), 1287–92.

17. L. E. Quint, G. M. Glazer, M. B. Orringer, and B. H. Gross. Esophageal carcinoma: CT findings. *Radiology*, **155** (1985), 171–5.

18. J. F. Griffith, J. Kew, A. C. Chan, and C. Metreweli. 3D CT imaging of oesophageal carcinoma. *Eur J Radiol*, **32** (1999), 216–20.

19. M. Coulomb, J. F. Lebas, R. Sarrazin, and M. Geindre. [Oesophageal cancer extension. Diagnostic contribution and effects on therapy of computed tomography. Report on 40 cases (author's trans.)]. *J Radiol*, **62** (1981), 475–87.

20. S. Rankin. The role of computerized tomography in the staging of oesophageal cancer. *Clin Radiol*, **42** (1990), 152–3.

21. J. Wayman, S. Chakraverty, S. M. Griffin, *et al*. Evaluation of local invasion by oesophageal carcinoma – a prospective study of prone computed tomography scanning. *Postgrad Med J*, **77** (2001), 181–4.

22. D. Picus, D. M. Balfe, R. E. Koehler, C. L. Roper, and J. W. Owen. Computed tomography in the staging of esophageal carcinoma. *Radiology*, **146** (1983), 433–8.

23. S. Takashima, N. Takeuchi, H. Shiozaki, *et al*. Carcinoma of the esophagus: CT vs MR imaging in determining resectability. *AJR Am J Roentgenol*, **156** (1991), 297–302.

24. L. Lehr, N. Rupp, and J. R. Siewert. Assessment of resectability of esophageal cancer by computed tomography and magnetic resonance imaging. *Surgery*, **103** (1988), 344–50.

25. H. S. Saunders, N. T. Wolfman, and D. J. Ott. Esophageal cancer. Radiologic staging. *Radiol Clin North Am*, **35** (1997), 281–94.

26. B. Kumbasar. Carcinoma of esophagus: radiologic diagnosis and staging. *Eur J Radiol*, **42** (2002), 170–80.

27. D. M. Balfe, M. A. Mauro, R. E. Koehler, *et al*. Gastrohepatic ligament: normal and pathologic CT anatomy. *Radiology*, **150** (1984), 485–90.

28. W. Schroder, S. E. Baldus, S. P. Monig, *et al.* Lymph node staging of esophageal squamous cell carcinoma in patients with and without neoadjuvant radiochemotherapy: histomorphologic analysis. *World J Surg*, **26** (2002), 584–7.

29. L. F. Wu, B. Z. Wang, J. L. Feng, *et al.* Preoperative TN staging of esophageal cancer: comparison of miniprobe ultrasonography, spiral CT and MRI. *World J Gastroenterol*, **9** (2003), 219–24.

30. Y. C. Yoon, K. S. Lee, Y. M. Shim, *et al.* Metastasis to regional lymph nodes in patients with esophageal squamous cell carcinoma: CT versus FDG PET for presurgical detection prospective study. *Radiology*, **227** (2003), 764–70.

31. H. Kato, T. Miyazaki, M. Nakajima, *et al.* The incremental effect of positron emission tomography on diagnostic accuracy in the initial staging of esophageal carcinoma. *Cancer*, **103** (2005), 148–56.

32. J. Romagnuolo, J. Scott, R. H. Hawes, *et al.* Helical CT versus EUS with fine needle aspiration for celiac nodal assessment in patients with esophageal cancer. *Gastrointest Endosc*, **55** (2002), 648–54.

33. C. Valls, E. Lopez, A. Guma, *et al.* Helical CT versus CT arterial portography in the detection of hepatic metastasis of colorectal carcinoma. *AJR Am J Roentgenol*, **170** (1998), 1341–7.

34. K. Kinkel, Y. Lu, M. Both, R. S. Warren, and R. F. Thoeni. Detection of hepatic metastases from cancers of the gastrointestinal tract by using noninvasive imaging methods (US, CT, MR imaging, PET): a meta-analysis. *Radiology*, **224** (2002), 748–56.

35. M. J. Gollub, R. Lefkowitz, C. S. Moskowitz, *et al.* Pelvic CT in patients with esophageal cancer. *AJR Am J Roentgenol*, **184** (2005), 487–90.

36. R. A. Halvorsen, Jr., K. Magruder-Habib, W. L. Foster, Jr., *et al.* Esophageal cancer staging by CT: long-term follow-up study. *Radiology*, **161** (1986), 147–51.

37. E. C. Unger, L. Coia, R. Gatenby, *et al.* CT staging of esophageal carcinoma in patients treated by primary radiation therapy and chemotherapy. *J Comput Assist Tomogr*, **16** (1992), 235–9.

38. F. L. Ampil, G. Caldito, B. D. Li, and R. Pelser. Computed tomographic staging of esophageal cancer and prognosis. *Radiat Med*, **19** (2001), 127–9.

39. L. E. Quint, G. M. Glazer, and M. B. Orringer. Esophageal imaging by MR and CT: study of normal anatomy and neoplasms. *Radiology*, **156** (1985), 727–31.

40. W. M. Thompson. Esophageal carcinoma. *Abdom Imaging*, **22** (1997), 138–42.

41. C. E. Reed and M. A. Eloubeidi. New techniques for staging esophageal cancer. *Surg Clin North Am*, **82** (2002), 697–710, v.

42. C. P. Hansen, K. Oskarsson, and D. Mortensen. Computed tomography for staging of oesophageal cancer. *Ann Chir Gynaecol*, **89** (2000), 14–18.

43. P. Buenaventura and J. D. Luketich. Surgical staging of esophageal cancer. *Chest Surg Clin N Am*, **10** (2000), 487–97.

44. M. B. Wallace, P. J. Nietert, C. Earle, *et al.* An analysis of multiple staging management strategies for carcinoma of the esophagus: computed tomography, endoscopic ultrasound, positron emission tomography, and thoracoscopy/laparoscopy. *Ann Thorac Surg*, **74** (2002), 1026–32.

45. A. B. Miller, B. Hoogstraten, M. Staquet, and A. Winkler. Reporting results of cancer treatment. *Cancer*, **47** (1981), 207–14.

46. S. J. Walker, S. M. Allen, A. Steel, M. H. Cullen, and H. R. Matthews. Assessment of the response to chemotherapy in oesophageal cancer. *Eur J Cardiothorac Surg*, **5** (1991), 519–22.

47. J. F. Griffith, A. C. Chan, L. T. Chow, *et al*. Assessing chemotherapy response of squamous cell oesophageal carcinoma with spiral CT. *Br J Radiol*, **72** (1999), 678–84.

48. A. J. Beer, H. A. Wieder, F. Lordick, *et al*. Adenocarcinomas of esophagogastric junction: multi-detector row CT to evaluate early response to neoadjuvant chemotherapy. *Radiology*, **239** (2006), 472–80.

49. M. A. Eloubeidi, A. C. Mason, R. A. Desmond, and H. B. El-Serag. Temporal trends (1973–1997) in survival of patients with esophageal adenocarcinoma in the United States: a glimmer of hope? *Am J Gastroenterol*, **98** (2003), 1627–33.

50. T. Iizuka, K. Isono, T. Kakegawa, and H. Watanabe. Parameters linked to ten-year survival in Japan of resected esophageal carcinoma. Japanese Committee for Registration of Esophageal Carcinoma Cases. *Chest*, **96** (1989), 1005–11.

51. C. Mariette, J. M. Balon, G. Piessen, *et al*. Pattern of recurrence following complete resection of esophageal carcinoma and factors predictive of recurrent disease. *Cancer*, **97** (2003), 1616–23.

52. J. G. Carlisle, L. E. Quint, I. R. Francis, *et al*. Recurrent esophageal carcinoma: CT evaluation after esophagectomy. *Radiology*, **189** (1993), 271–5.

53. H. U. Kauczor, P. Mildenberger, F. Schweden, A. Heintz, and H. H. Schild. [Patterns of recurrence of esophageal carcinoma after esophageal resection and gastric interposition: CT findings]. *Rofo*, **161** (1994), 113–19.

54. M. Morita, H. Kuwano, S. Ohno, M. Furusawa, and K. Sugimachi. Characteristics and sequence of the recurrent patterns after curative esophagectomy for squamous cell carcinoma. *Surgery*, **116** (1994), 1–7.

55. A. Katayama, K. Mafune, Y. Tanaka, *et al*. Autopsy findings in patients after curative esophagectomy for esophageal carcinoma. *J Am Coll Surg*, **196** (2003), 866–73.

56. C. D. Becker, P. A. Barbier, F. Terrier, and B. Porcellini. Patterns of recurrence of esophageal carcinoma after transhiatal esophagectomy and gastric interposition. *AJR Am J Roentgenol*, **148** (1987), 273–7.

57. M. Kantarci, P. Polat, F. Alper, *et al*. Comparison of CT and MRI for the diagnosis recurrent esophageal carcinoma after operation. *Dis Esophagus*, **17** (2004), 32–7.

6

FDG-PET and PET/CT in Esophageal Cancer

Sheila C. Rankin

Introduction

The anatomical imaging techniques of computer tomography (CT) and endo-scopic ultrasound (EUS) have limitations in the staging of esophageal cancer, in assessing response to therapy, and in predicting survival. Functional imaging using positron emission tomography (PET) has been shown to provide unique informa-tion in other tumors and is increasingly being used in oesophageal cancer.

Positron emission tomography

PET is an imaging technique that can map functional activity before structural changes have taken place and has established a recognized place in imaging cancer. The most commonly used isotope at the present time is ^{18}F-fluoro-2-deoxy-D-glucose (FDG), which can differentiate malignant from normal tissue based on the enhanced glucose transport and glycolysis exhibited by many tumor cells. FDG is a glucose analogue, and both FDG and glucose are taken up by cells via the membrane glucose transporter system and are phosphorylated by hexokinase. Unlike glucose, FDG-6-phosphate does not cross the cell membrane and is trapped in cells and is visualized. It can be dephosphorylated, but this is a slow process particularly in cancer cells that lack or have reduced levels of glucose-6-phosphatase. FDG accumulation depends on the rate of transport through the cell membrane that is mediated by glucose transporters (GLUT). Many malignant cells, including gastrointestinal tumors, show increased expression of GLUT-1, contributing to increased FDG accumulation, and this corre-lates with tumor invasiveness and poor survival in some cancers. Cancers cells, including esophageal cancer, may also show increased levels of activity of hexokinase

Carcinoma of the Esophagus, ed. Sheila C. Rankin. Published by Cambridge University Press. © Cambridge University Press 2008.

and therefore increased uptake of FDG. Increased blood flow or hypoxia associated with tumors may also increase FDG uptake [1,2].

Following intravenous injection FDG is continuously accumulated in metabolizing cells. More than 40 minutes after injection the uptake of FDG in cells is proportional to its glucose utilization with more uptake seen in viable tumor cells than in necrotic tissue, but FDG uptake is also seen in inflammatory tissue. An intravenous injection of 300–400 MBq of FDG is used in most institutions and the patient is imaged at least 1 h after injection. Delaying the time of imaging may improve the tumor to background ratio, although radioactive decay may decrease the image quality. High glucose levels interfere with tumor targeting via competitive inhibition of FDG uptake by glucose, and although an elevated glucose does not preclude PET imaging, the tumor to background ratio may be reduced.

Attenuation correction is performed both to improve anatomic localization and to quantify the uptake. The commonest method of quantification is the standardized uptake value (SUV), which is the ratio of injected activity to body weight (concentration of radioactivity in the tumor (MBq/ml) × patient body weight (g)/ injected dose (MBq)). Although the SUV can be compared in the same patient on the same scanner with standard imaging protocols, the same values cannot necessarily be applied in all units.

The spatial resolution of the present FDG-PET systems is 5–8 mm. Lesions smaller that 1 cm may therefore not be resolved fully and tracer concentrations will be underestimated because of the partial volume effect; however, if the concentration of FDG is high enough, lesions less than 1 cm will be detected.

The development of the fusion of multidetector CT and a positron emission scanner in PET/CT is now widely available. This combination allows the low-dose CT to be used for attenuation correction with a decrease in overall scan time, but with an increase in radiation dose to the patient, and also accurate anatomic coregistration as the patient does not move between the two acquisitions. PET/ CT has a higher diagnostic accuracy than PET alone in esophageal cancer and decreases the number of futile surgical procedures by detecting occult metastases [3,4]. Bar-Shalom *et al.* [5] compared PET/CT, with PET reviewed side by side with CT to assess detection, accuracy of localization, and characterization of malignant sites in patients with esophageal cancer. PET/CT provided incremental value in 22% (25 of 115 sites), and PET/CT was more specific and accurate than PET alone for detection of sites of disease (81 and 90% versus 59 and 83%, respectively).

Staging

The prognosis for esophageal cancer is poor, and up to 50% of the patients present with advanced disease with multiple sites of nodal involvement or distant metastases. Patients with limited disease can be treated with surgery either initially or following induction chemoradiotherapy (CRT). The surgical choices include esophageal resection via a transthoracic approach with two- or three-field lymphadenectomy or transhiatal resection, but patients with distant metastases are not surgical candidates and should be treated with CRT. Accurate staging using the TNM classification is therefore important in order to suggest the most appropriate treatment and to offer prognostic information.

T stage

Squamous cell carcinoma (SCC) and adenocarcinoma of the esophagus both demonstrate high avidity for FDG [6,7,8], although SCC more so than adenocarcinoma. False positives will occur with esophagitis, either peptic or infective, and also in patients with strictures that have been dilated. False-negative results occur in small tumors, which is partly a reflection of the limited spatial resolution of the present generation of PET scanners.

Kato *et al.* [9] examined 149 consecutive patients at diagnosis, mainly with *SCC*, and identified the primary tumor in 80% overall. However, it did depend on the T stage, with 43% of T1 tumors (18% of pT1a and 61% of pT1b), 83% of pT2, 97% pT3, and 100% of pT4 tumors detected (Figure 6.1). Yoon *et al.* reported a sensitivity of 91% for the detection of squamous cell cancer with all the pT1 or pTis tumors missed [10].

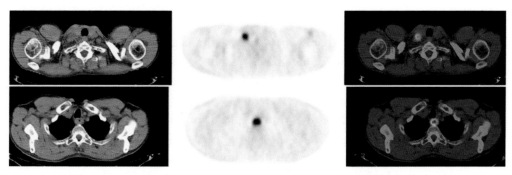

Figure 6.1 **FDG-PET of a patient with squamous cell carcinoma of the upper third of the esophagus. Uptake in small right supraclavicular node, which was not identified on the original staging CT scan.**

The sensitivity for the detection for *adenocarcinoma* is more variable particularly of the gastroesophageal junction and the proximal stomach. Even large-volume tumors may show no or little uptake in 17–20% of cases [11,12]. This low avidity appears to be related to the diffuse growth pattern and the degree of differentiation of the tumor, with poorly differentiated tumors less avid. In gastric adenocarcinoma Stahl *et al.* found low uptake in signet ring and mucinous carcinomas, with 67% of the mucinous adenocarcinomas visualized and only 25% of the signet ring [13]. The high false-negative rate may be related not only to the large quantities of metabolically inert mucin but also to the lack of expression of glucose transporters (GLUT-1) on the signet ring cells, whereas patients with SCC of the esophagus have been reported to have a high expression of GLUT-1 [14,15].

Although FDG-PET has a relatively high sensitivity in identifying the primary tumor, it is unable to differentiate the layers of the esophagus and establish the T stage. Flamen *et al.* studied a group of patients with both adenocarcinoma and SCC and found that FDG was 95% sensitive in the detection of the primary tumor with a mean SUV of 13.5, but there was no correlation between the SUV and the T stage at surgery [16].

Liberale *et al.* found no significant difference between PET and CT in the detection of the primary tumor (sensitivity 87% for PET and 84% for CT), although CT, with its superior spatial resolution, identified mediastinal invasion not seen on the PET scan and was better for local staging [17]. The combination of PET and CT may help in this regard but overall provides no additional advantage for the primary tumor [5].

Endoscopic ultrasound provides the most accurate T staging and is superior to both PET and CT, and although it may both overstage and understage patients, remains the best modality for the assessment of the T stage [16,18,19].

N stage

The oesophagus has a rich and chaotic nodal drainage that extends from the neck to the abdomen. The site of the primary is not a predictor of nodal involvement, with 12% of upper oesophageal tumors involving the abdomen and 27% of lower oesophageal tumors involving cervical nodes [20].

Nodal staging provides important prognostic information with a 5-year survival for node-negative patients of 42–72% as opposed to that of node-positive patients of 10–12% [21]. The number of nodes is important, and if more than four lymph nodes are involved, survival is similar to that of M1 disease [22,23], and the size of nodal deposit is an independent predictor of survival [24].

Despite the importance of nodal staging, the noninvasive cross-sectional techniques have well-known limitations. There are many studies assessing the accuracy of PET for local nodal metastases, and the results are very variable. The earlier studies produced good results. Flanagan *et al.* reported that PET was more sensitive and specific than CT (72 and 82% for PET versus 28 and 73% for CT) [7], and Kole *et al.* reported a sensitivity of 92% for local nodal detection [25]. The later studies produced different results, with some of the reported variability arising from the study methodology with mixed populations of adenocarcinoma and SCC and whether the correlation was with a two or three-field lymphadenectomy or transhiatal resection, which will identify fewer nodes and may understage the disease. Kim *et al.* studied 50 patients with SCC, all of whom underwent two or three-field lymphadenectomy and found PET more sensitive (52%) than CT (15%) with a similar specificity [8]. Yoon *et al.* studied 81 patients with SCC and full surgical correlation [10]. PET was more sensitive than CT for individual nodal groups (30 versus 11%) and also for nodal staging (64 versus 31%), but its specificity was less (68 versus 86%), with false positive results in hilar lymph nodes in patients with chronic lung disease or previous tuberculosis, and these authors concluded that neither test was sufficiently sensitive for the detection of local nodal disease. Kneist *et al.* were the only group to find CT more sensitive than PET but less specific (75 and 71% versus 42 and 94%, respectively) [26]; these authors thought FDG-PET provided no management advantage and should be reserved for patients with inconclusive CT findings.

Most institutions use the combination of CT and EUS for the assessment of the primary tumor and nodal disease, and the results of the comparison of PET with the combination of CT and EUS are conflicting. Choi *et al.* preformed a study in 48 patients with SCC and compared the results to EUS [27]; this group found PET better than CT for individual nodes (sensitivity 57%, specificity 97%, and accuracy 85% for PET, and 18, 99, and 78% for CT, respectively) and also to be more accurate for nodal staging than either CT or EUS (83% for PET, 60% for CT, and 58% for EUS). The poor results with EUS were attributed to incomplete examinations because of tight stenotic esophageal lesions. Lerut *et al.* looking at a group with both SCC and adenocarcinoma found that CT/EUS was more sensitive but less specific than PET for locoregional nodes (sensitivity 83%, specificity 45%, and accuracy 69% for EUS/CT versus 22, 91, and 48% for PET, respectively) [28]. Rasanen *et al.* who studied patients with adenocarcinoma also found EUS to be the most sensitive test for local nodal disease, with PET the most specific (89 and 54% versus 37 and 100%) [12]. Much better results were obtained by Lowe *et al.* who found that PET had a sensitivity of 82%, with CT, PET, and EUS comparable for both sensitivity and specificity [18].

van Westreenen *et al.* in a systematic review of the literature looking at pooled data for locoregional nodes found that the sensitivity for PET is 0.51 (95% CI 0.34–0.69) with a specificity of 0.84 (95% CI 0.76–0.91) [29]. Overall, the diagnostic accuracy for FDG-PET for nodal disease in esophageal cancer appears to be lower than in other tumors such as non-small-cell lung cancer. False negatives may be related either to small volume disease or to the obscuration of nodes in close proximity to the primary tumor by uptake within the tumor (Figure 6.2). The false-positive results include misinterpretation of physiologic uptake, for example, in brown fat and skeletal muscle. Some of these problems will be overcome with PET/CT with its superior anatomic resolution. Yuan *et al.* compared the results of PET with those of PET/CT and found that there was an increase in sensitivity, specificity, and accuracy with PET/CT for nodal staging (sensitivity 81%, specificity 87%, and accuracy 86% for PET versus 93, 92, and 92% for PET/CT, respectively) [30].

Despite the importance of nodal staging in management, there appears to be no one noninvasive test that is both sensitive and specific for locoregional nodes. FDG-PET will always have limitations in nodes close to the primary but is of more value for other regional nodes, and EUS with fine-needle cytology holds most potential, as the results are independent of nodal size [31].

Metastases

Patients with distant metastases in either lymph nodes or solid organs have a very poor outcome and should not undergo surgical resection. Patients with only local disease have a 60% 30-month survival, whereas if distant metastases are present, the survival is only 20% [32]. The commonest sites of metastatic disease are in non-regional lymph nodes, liver, lung, and bone. FDG-PET has been reported to be superior to CT in non-regional lymph nodes, as it identifies tumor in normal-sized lymph nodes where uptake is not obscured by uptake in adjacent tumor, and enlarged reactive nodes may show no increased FDG uptake. False-positive results occur in inflammatory processes including sarcoidosis and chronic lung diseases. Kinkel *et al.* compared CT, US, MRI, and PET for the detection of liver metastases from gastrointestinal tumors [33], and using a specificity of 85%, the sensitivity of CT was 63%, US 55%, PET 90%, and MRI 76%, respectively, although a more recent study by Selzner *et al.* found that contrast-enhanced multidetector CT and

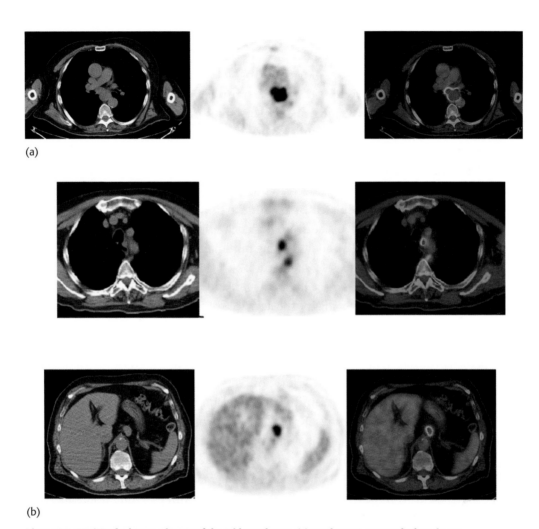

Figure 6.2 PET/CT of adenocarcinoma of the mid esophagus. (a) On the FDG-PET study the primary tumor is difficult to separate from the adjacent subcarinal nodes, but it easily identified as separate on the PET/CT. (b) Same patient demonstrating positive celiac nodes and uptake in small mediastinal nodes.

PET/CT produced very similar results in patients with liver metastases from colonic carcinoma [34]. Kato *et al.* found FDG-PET was superior to isotope bone scans particularly for lytic metastases (sensitivity 92% and specificity 93% for PET versus 77 and 84% for isotope bone scans, respectively) [35], and Taira *et al.* found PET/CT had a positive predictive value of 95% when PET and CT findings were concordant, although there was a marked decrease in PPV when the results were discordant [36]. Flamen *et al.* compared FDG-PET, CT, and EUS and found that the diagnostic accuracy for metastatic disease was 82% for PET and 64%

for EUS and CT combined, mainly because of the superior sensitivity of PET (74 versus 47%) [16]. Similar results were reported by Lerut *et al.*, with upstaging in 15% and downstaging in 7% of patients [37]. However, Lowe *et al.* found that the results for the three investigations were very similar [18], perhaps because in this study all PET-positive lesions underwent biopsy for confirmation. This group looked at the treatment assignment and found that although the results were similar the tests were complementary, with EUS most useful for locoregional disease and CT and PET more useful for the assessment of distant disease.

The sensitivity of FDG-PET decreases with decreasing size of tumor, with lesions less than 1 cm often difficult to visualize due to the partial volume effect although if they are very avid they will be seen. Luketich *et al.* studied 87 patients prior to surgery and compared PET and CT using minimally invasive surgery (laparoscopy and thoracoscopy) as the gold standard [32]. FDG-PET was superior to CT and identified 69% of lesions, missing lung, liver, and peritoneal metastases that were all less than 1 cm, giving a diagnostic accuracy of 84%. In this study CT was 46% sensitive, with an overall accuracy of 63%. Blackstock *et al.* found occult metastases in 40% of their patients with locally advanced esophageal cancer [38]. Those patients who were upstaged with FDG-PET had a poor prognosis, with a 2-year survival of 17% compared to 64% for those without occult metastases. Duong *et al.* found FDG-PET was more sensitive and specific than EUS and CT for distant metastases, with discordant results in 44% of patients, FDG-PET upstaging in 26% and downstaging in 18%, and incremental treatment change in 32% [39].

Stahl *et al.* found that reading PET and CT together reduced the false-positive rate for PET from 10 to 3%, with PET changing management in 15% [40]. This is in agreement with the early studies comparing PET with PET/CT, where PET/CT had an incremental value over PET alone of 22%, improving anatomic localization and characterization of lesions, with a significant change in patient management in 10% [5,41].

There are an increasing number of studies on the effectiveness of PET in staging esophageal cancer, and its main impact appears to be in the detection of occult metastases. van Westreenen undertook a retrospective review of 203 patients assessing the impact of preoperative staging on exploratory surgery [42]. Resection was abandoned in 38% because of distant metastases in 29% and locally advanced disease in 9%, and FDG-PET was the only modality that predicted curative surgery. However, as false-positive results may occur with inflammatory or infective processes, histologic confirmation will be required if there will be a significant change to patient management [43,44].

Wallace and coworkers have compared the effectiveness of different strategies for the preoperative assessment of esophageal cancer based on life expectancy, prevalence of disease, cost of procedures, and the probability of death from minimally invasive procedures [45]. These authors concluded that the combination of CT with EUS with fine-needle aspiration cytology (FNAC) was the most inexpensive and offered more quality-adjusted life years. PET + EUS + FNAC was slightly more effective but more expensive. The development of PET/CT combined with EUS and FNAC would appear to be the best option but would also be more expensive.

Overall, the evidence indicates that FDG-PET should be performed prior to any therapy undertaken with curative intent to exclude occult metastases [46].

Prognosis

In patients who undergo curative surgery without CRT, the number and location of positive nodes and whether there is extracapsular spread influences survival [8,47], and in those patients who receive preoperative CRT the posttreatment staging, particularly the number of nodes and the size of the metatastatic deposit, are independent prognostic factors for overall survival [9,48].

The advantage of FDG-PET in providing prognostic information has been demonstrated by several authors. Choi *et al.* using multivariate analysis found that the tumor length and the number of positive nodes on FDG-PET were independent significant prognostic predictors of overall survival in patients with SCC, with the number of PET positive nodes predicting both disease-free interval and overall survival [49].

Cerfolio *et al.* found the maximum SUV (SUV_{max}) was an independent predictor of survival, with a 4-year survival of 89% in patients with a maximum SUV of 6.6 or less, whereas it was 31% in those with an SUV_{max} of greater than 6.6 [50]. Rizk *et al.* using an SUV_{max} of 4.5 found patients with an SUV_{max} less than this had a 3-year survival of 95%, whereas if the SUV_{max} was greater than 4.5, the 3-year survival was 57%, and the survival advantage of an SUV_{max} value of 4.5 or less was seen within different groups according to T stage [51]. Not all authors agree and Stahl *et al.* found no correlation between the SUV and survival or tumor-free survival [40].

Treatment planning

Recently, FDG-PET has been integrated into radiotherapy planning since functional images allow better delineation of the anatomical extent of the tumor and associated lymphadenopathy. Vrieze *et al.* undertook a retrospective study of 30 patients to determine the additional value of FDG-PET in the delineation of the clinical target volume [52]. The lymph nodes were scored on conventional (EUS and CT) and functional imaging, and the effect of discordant results on the radiation field was assessed. There were discordant findings in 47%. In 10% of patients FDG-PET would have increased the irradiated volume and in 10% the volume would have been decreased. These authors suggested that as the chance of a false negative with FDG-PET is not negligible the volume should not be decreased if the conventional imaging is positive, but if the FDG-PET is positive, the volume should be increased even if conventional imaging is negative. Leong *et al.* compared PET/CT with CT for radiotherapy planning [53]. These authors assumed PET/CT would more accurately demonstrate the full extent of disease and found that PET/CT altered the clinical extent of tumor in 38%, identifying both distant metastases and unsuspected regional disease. Radiotherapy planning with CT alone would have excluded PET-positive disease in 69%, with the main difference being in defining the tumor length. Moureau-Zabotto *et al.* found that the addition of FDG-PET increased the gross tumor volume in 21% and decreased it in 35% of their patients [54]. There was also a modification in the delineation of the gross tumor volume, with an alteration in the total lung volume irradiated in 74%, dose reduction in 12%, and dose increase in 13%. Konski *et al.* integrated FDG-PET and EUS in the CT planning [55]. In this study the length of the tumor was significantly longer on CT than on EUS or FDG-PET, and EUS identified more celiac and periesophageal nodes compared with FDG-PET and CT. Both EUS and PET can provide additional information to aid in the precise delineation of the gross tumor volume.

Response assessment

The prognosis for locally advanced esophageal disease is poor (median survival 3–5 months), and the best option for cure in locally advanced disease is radical surgery, but the long-term survival is still poor with frequent recurrences, suggesting that tumors are being understaged by conventional imaging. Therefore, preoperative multimodality therapy with chemotherapy with or without radiotherapy is now being used in an attempt to improve surgical results with the aim of eradicating lymphatic or hematogenous metastases, to improve survival and reduce local recurrence [56,57], and also to shrink the primary tumor to improve resectabilty. Patients who receive maximum benefit from neoadjuvant chemotherapy are those who have a complete pathologic response, which occurs in 15–30% of patients, and this group have a 3-year survival of 60% [58]. Korst *et al.* found that patients who responded to CRT had a 5-year survival of 63% compared with the 5-year survival of 23% in the nonresponders, suggesting responders represent a group that may benefit from surgery following neoadjuvant therapy [59]. Levine *et al.* demonstrated the predictive value of FDG-PET in identifying responders [60]. In their group of patients who underwent preoperative CRT 27% had a complete response and 14.5% had residual microscopic disease. A pretreatment SUV of more than 15 was associated with a significant response in 77.8% of patients (complete and/or microscopic residual), whereas if the pretreatment SUV was less than 15, only 24.4% had such a response. A decrease in SUV of more than 10 following treatment was also associated with a significant response in 71% of patients, compared with a response of only 33% if the decrease in SUV was less than 10.

However, in 15–19% of patients there will be disease progression during the neoadjuvant therapy, and these patients do not benefit from the therapy, may suffer toxic side effects, and the surgery might be delayed and no longer be appropriate. In nonresponders survival is similar or worse after resection than in those patients who undergo surgery without neoadjuvant therapy, with the nonresponders having a greater postoperative mortality and morbidity. Therefore, it would be helpful to identify tumor response early in therapy, and in nonresponders other treatment options including a change in chemotherapy, addition of radiotherapy, or immediate surgery may be more appropriate.

Response to therapy is evaluated using the conventional imaging of CT and EUS. Both of these modalities have difficulty differentiating viable tumor from posttherapy necrosis and fibrosis, and the delay between cell death and tumor shrinkage may influence any measurements (Figure 6.3). Alterations in metabolic activity in response to therapy precede anatomic change, and FDG-PET has been shown to be sensitive in imaging response to therapy in many other malignancies [61,62,63]. In an initial study by Weber *et al.* of patients with esophageal cancer FDG-PET was undertaken before and 14 days after commencing cisplatin-based chemotherapy [64]. Using an SUV reduction of 35% to indicate a response, this group found metabolic response predicted a histopathologic response and was associated with an improved survival (50 months). In a larger study the same group found the metabolic responders showed a major histopathologic response rate (<10% viable cells remaining) of 44% and a 3-year survival of 70%, whereas the nonresponders had a histopathologic response rate of only 5% with a 3-year survival of 35% [65]. In this study, in those patients who had a successful resection, using multivariate analysis metabolic response was the only factor predicting recurrence. Wieder *et al.*

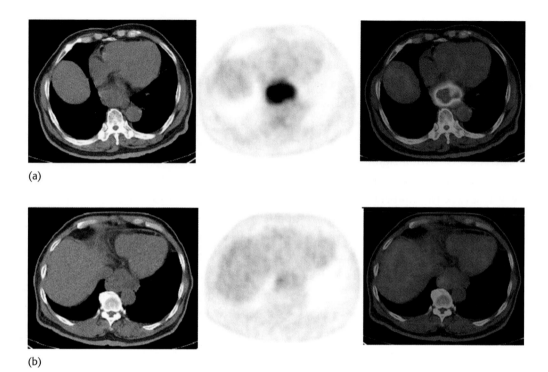

(a)

(b)

Figure 6.3 Response to therapy. (a) Staging PET/CT pre treatment. (b) Postchemotherapy. The size of the tumor is virtually unchanged on the CT scan but has shown a complete metabolic response following chemotherapy.

performed an initial FDG-PET followed by one 14 days after the commencement of chemotherapy and one on completion of chemotherapy in patients with adenocarcinoma and found no correlation between the decreased FDG uptake and the tumor size based on CT at 14 days [66], but the FDG reduction did correlate with tumor size on completion of therapy, indicating that metabolic response was a more sensitive indicator than tumor size in predicting response. This group undertook a similar study in patients with SCC who underwent FDG-PET before, 2 weeks after induction chemo/radiotherapy, and again prior to surgery. They found a significant difference in the SUV decreased between the responders (44 ± 15%) and the nonresponders (21 ± 14%), with the changes in metabolic activity after 14 days being more specific for response than the changes at completion of therapy [67].

However, Gillham *et al.* studied 32 patients, predominantly with adenocarcinoma, before and 1 week after commencement of CRT and obtained rather different results [68]. This group found no significant difference in the reduction in SUV between the responders and nonresponders and suggested that radiotherapy, which causes an inflammatory reaction, may mask the SUV reduction in responders. They suggested that perhaps early assessment with FDG-PET for response assessment should be limited to patients undergoing chemotherapy without radiotherapy.

Other groups have looked at response assessment at the end of treatment prior to resection. Flamen *et al.* found FDG-PET to be both sensitive and specific (71 and 82%, respectively) in identifying a major response [69], although response was both overestimated and underestimated in 11%. This group also found the metabolic response was a strong predictor for survival (median survival 16.3 months in responders versus 6.4 months in nonresponders). Brucher *et al.* studied a group of patients with SCC before and 3 weeks after neoadjuvant CRT prior to surgery [70]. In responders the SUV decreased by $72 \pm 11\%$, but by only $42 \pm 22\%$ in nonresponders. Using a threshold of a 52% decrease in SUV, the sensitivity to detect response was 100% with a specificity of 55%.

Westerterp *et al.* undertook a systematic review of CT, EUS, and FDG-PET in assessing response to therapy, with receiver operating characteristic (ROC) analysis used to summarize and compare the diagnostic accuracy of the three methods [71]. The sensitivity for CT, EUS, and FDG-PET ranged from 33 to 55%, 50 to 100%, and 71 to 100%, respectively, and the specificity ranged from 50 to71%, 36 to 100%, and 55 to 100%, respectively. Overall, the accuracy for CT was much less than for EUS and FDG-PET, although in these studies single-slice systems were used and the results may be better with multidetector CT [72]. The results with EUS and FDG-PET were very similar, although in 20% of patients the EUS was either suboptimal or not feasible. There are some limitations to this review. The overall number of appropriate studies was small, and in none of the studies was there a direct comparison of the modalities within a single patient group; nevertheless, the authors concluded that FDG-PET was a promising noninvasive modality for assessing response, but larger studies with direct comparisons of the modalities are needed.

Swisher *et al.* compared CT, EUS, and FDG-PET in a group of 103 patients who underwent CRT prior to surgery [73]. Using post-CRT data, these authors developed thresholds for each modality to differentiate responders ($<10\%$ viable tumor remaining) from nonresponders and used a wall thickness greater than 14.5 mm for CT, tumor length greater than 1 cm for EUS, and an SUV greater than 4 in the primary for PET. Using these criteria, FDG-PET was more accurate (76%) than EUS (68%) or CT (62%). Only a post-CRT SUV greater than 4 was an independent predictor of survival, with a 2-year survival of 34% compared with a 2-year survival of 64% in patients with an SUV less than 4. None of the imaging modalities could accurately differentiate a complete responder (0% viable tumor) from microscopic residual disease (1–10% viable tumor), so a patient with a complete response on imaging could have some residual disease and may require further intervention.

Duong *et al.* reported similar findings in their study comparing FDG-PET with CT [74]. These authors found a complete metabolic response in 43% of the patients, whereas only 8% demonstrated a complete response using CT criteria. The 2-year survival in responders was 78 versus 33% in nonresponders. In this study the complete responders in whom resection was not performed had a comparable survival to those who underwent surgical resection, and these authors suggested that potentially a more conservative approach of no resection could be offered to those patients who had a complete metabolic response, with the proviso that these patients should have close follow-up to detect early local relapse.

Overall, FDG-PET does appear to hold most promise for the assessment of response, but a complete metabolic response does not exclude microscopic residual disease and the use of SUV data does have some problems, as this is not necessarily reproducible in different institutions.

Recurrent disease

The recurrence rate after resection is high (34–79%), with the majority of recurrences presenting within 1 year and nearly all within 2 years after primary surgery. Recurrences are classified as local or distant, with lymph node recurrence and hematogenous metastases to the lungs common [75,76]. The therapeutic options at this stage include radical or palliative re-resection, laser thermocoagulation, stenting, chemotherapy, brachytherapy or radiotherapy, and early detection and aggressive therapy may lead to prolonged tumor-free survival [77]. In approximately 30% of patients the recurrence is in the operative field, with lymph node involvement or mediastinal masses. FDG-PET is less influenced by anatomical distortion postsurgery or radiotherapy than the other imaging modalities and should be helpful in these cases.

Flamen *et al.* in a study of patients with clinical or radiological suspected recurrence compared FDG-PET with the conventional workup of CT and EUS [78]. In this study all equivocal lesions on any modality were called positive. The sensitivity for FDG-PET for periesophageal recurrence was 100% with a specificity of 57% and accuracy of 74%, whereas the conventional workup was 100% sensitive, 93%

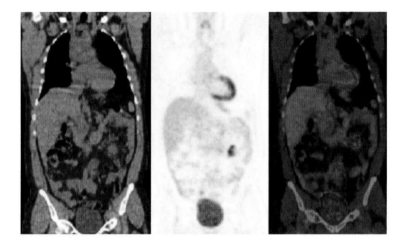

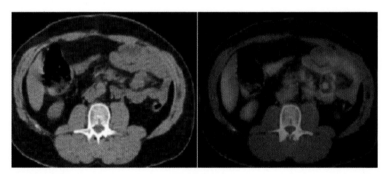

Figure 6.4 Recurrent tumor within the peritoneum – not identified as separate from the bowel on the original CT.

specific, and 96% accurate. The false positives on FDG-PET were found in those patients who had stenotic lesions that had undergone repeated dilatations. The majority of recurrences were distant metastases, and for the diagnosis of regional and distant recurrence the sensitivity, specificity, and accuracy of FDG-PET compared with conventional imaging was 94, 82, and 87% versus 81, 82, and 81%, respectively (Figure 6.4). Although in this study there was no significant difference in the results between the methods of investigation, on a patient basis FDG-PET did provide additional information in 11 out of 41 patients (27%), identifying unsuspected recurrence in 5 and upstaging in a further 5 patients.

Kato *et al.* looked at a group of postsurgical patients, only 8% of whom were symptomatic, but 35% had recurrent disease [79]. FDG-PET was 100% sensitive, but only 75% specific for local recurrence compared to CT (84 and 86%, respectively). FDG-PET may be more sensitive than CT for local recurrence, as CT may fail to differentiate postoperative changes from recurrent tumors. The false positives for FDG-PET were in physiological uptake in the gastric tube and in mediastinal lymph nodes probably related to chronic lung disease. For distant recurrence the diagnostic accuracy for FDG-PET and CT were similar for liver metastases, whereas FDG-PET was less sensitive than CT (50 versus 100%) for lung metastases, mainly because of the limited spatial resolution for FDG-PET where small metastases less than 1 cm may not be identified. FDG-PET was more sensitive for bone metastases (100 versus 17%, respectively), partly because a whole body image was obtained with PET and half of the metastases were outside the regions included in the CT scan. Zhang *et al.* found that PET/CT was significantly more sensitive, specific, and accurate than CT alone (97.7, 100, and 85.7% versus 77.3, 61.7, and 78.6%, respectively) for recurrent disease [80].

Conclusion

The role of FDG-PET is established in many malignancies, and PET/CT provides additional benefits. FDG-PET is now becoming more important in the management of esophageal cancer, as it can distinguish between benign and malignant disease, assess the stage of the disease, detect tumor recurrence, and perhaps more importantly both monitor and predict response to therapy. It is also increasingly being used to define radiotherapy portals, and future developments will include utilization of other ligands to assess hypoxia, cell death, and protein metabolism [61].

REFERENCES

1. T. Fukunaga, S. Okazumi, Y. Koide, *et al.* Evaluation of esophageal cancers using fluorine-18-fluorodeoxyglucose PET. *J Nucl Med*, **39** (1998), 1002–7.
2. J. Czernin and M. E. Phelps. Positron emission tomography scanning: current and future applications. *Annu Rev Med*, **53** (2002), 89–112.
3. L. Rampin, C. Nani, S. Fanti, *et al.* Value of PET-CT fusion imaging in avoiding potential pitfalls in the interpretation of [18] F-FDG accumulation in the distal oesophagus. *Eur J Nucl Med Mol Imaging*, **32** (2005), 990–2.
4. R. F. Muden, H. A. Macapiniac, and J. J. Erasmus. Esophageal cancer: the role of integrated CT-PET in initial staging and response assessment after preoperative therapy. *J Thorac Imaging*, **21** (2006), 137–45.

5. R. Bar-Shalom, L. Guralnik, M. Tsalic, *et al.* The additional value of PET/CT over PET in FDG imaging of oesophageal cancer. *Eur J Nucl Med Mol Imaging*, **32** (2005), 918–24.

6. S. Rankin, H. Taylor, G. Cook, *et al.* Computed tomography and positron emission tomography in the pre-operative staging of oesophageal carcinoma. *Clin Radiol*, **53** (1998), 659–65.

7. F. L. Flanagan, F. Dehdashti, B. A. Siegal, *et al.* staging of esophageal cancer with 18F-fluorodeoxyglucose positron emission tomography. *Am J Roentgenol*, **168** (1997), 417–24.

8. K. Kim, S. J. Park, B. T. Kim, K. S. Lee, and Y. M. Shim. Evaluation of lymph node metastases in squamous cell carcinoma of the esophagus with positron emission tomography. *Ann Thorac Surg*, **71** (2001), 290–4.

9. H. Kato, T. Miyazaki, M. Nakajima, *et al.* The incremental effect of positron emission tomography on diagnostic accuracy in the initial staging of esophageal carcinoma. *Cancer*, **103** (2005), 148–56.

10. Y. C. Yoon, K. S. Lee, Y. M. Shim, *et al.* Metastasis to regional lymph nodes in patients with esophageal squamous cell carcinoma: CT vs FDG PET for presurgical detection – prospective study. *Radiology*, **227** (2003), 764–70.

11. P. Flamen, T. Lerut, K. Haustermans, E. Van Cutsem, and L. Mortelmans. Position of positron emission tomography and other imaging diagnostic modalities in esophageal cancer. *Q J Nucl Med Mol Imaging*, **48** (2004), 96–108.

12. J. V. Rasanen, E. I. Sihvo, M. J. Knuuti, *et al.* Prospective analysis of accuracy of positron emission tomography, computed tomography, and endoscopic ultrasonography in staging of adenocarcinoma of the esophagus and esophagogastric junction. *Ann Surg Oncol*, **10** (2003), 954–60.

13. A. Stahl, K. Ott, W. A. Weber, *et al.* FDG PET imaging of locally advanced gastric carcinomas: correlation with endoscopic and histopathological findings. *Eur J Nucl Med Mol Imaging*, **30** (2003), 288–95.

14. T. Kawamura, T. Kusakabe, T. Sugino, *et al.* Expression of glucose transporter-1 in human gastric carcinoma: Association with tumour aggressiveness, metastases and patient survival. *Cancer*, **92** (2001), 634–41.

15. K. H. Takita, T. Myazaki, M. Nakajima, *et al.* Correlation of 18-F-fluorodeoxyglucose (FDG) accumulation with glucose transporter (Glut-1) expression in esophageal squamous cell carcinoma. *Anticancer Res*, **23** (2003), 3263–72.

16. P. Flamen, T. Lerut, E. Van Cutsem, *et al.* Utility of positron emission tomography for the staging of patients with potentially operable esophageal carcinoma. *J Clin Oncol*, **18** (2000), 3202–10.

17. G. Liberale, J. L. Van Laethem, F. Gay, *et al.* The role of PET scan in the preoperative management of oesophageal cancer. *Eur J Surg Oncol*, **30** (2004), 942–7.

18. V. J. Lowe, F. Booya, J. G. Fletcher, *et al.* Comparison of positron emission tomography, computed tomography and endoscopic ultrasound in the initial staging of patients with esophageal cancer. *Mol Imaging Biol*, **7** (2005), 422–30.

19. S. Kelly, K. M. Harris, E. Berry, *et al.* A systematic review of the staging performance of endoscopic ultrasound in gastro-oesophageal carcinoma. *Gut*, **49** (2001), 534–9.

20. H. Akiyama, M. Tsurumaru, H. Udagawa, and Y. Kajiyama. Radical lymph node dissection for cancer of the thoracic esophagus. *Ann Surg*, **220** (1994), 364–73.

21. T. Lerut, W. Coosemans, G. Decker, *et al.* Cancer of the esophagus and gastr-esophageal junction: Potentially curative therapies. *Surg Oncol*, **10** (2001), 113–22.

22. M. A. Eloubeidi, R. Desmond, M. R. Arguedas, C. E. Reed, and C. M. Wilcox. Prognostic factors for the survival of patients with esophageal carcinoma in the U.S.: the importance of tumor length and lymph node status. *Cancer*, **95** (2002), 1434–43.

23. N. Rizk, E. Venkatraman, B. Park, *et al.* The prognostic importance of the number of involved lymph nodes in esophageal cancer: implications for revisions of the American Joint Committee on Cancer staging system. *J Thorac Cardiovasc Surg*, **132** (2006), 1374–81.

24. T. Komori, Y. Doki, T. Kabuto, *et al.* Prognostic significance of the size of cancer nests in metastatic lymph nodes in human esophageal cancers. *J Surg Oncol*, **82** (2003), 19–27.

25. A. C. Kole, J. T. Plukker, O. E. Nieweg, and W. Vaalburg. Positron emission tomography for staging of esophageal and gastroesophageal malignancy. *Br J Cancer*, **78** (1998), 521–7.

26. W. Kneist, M. Schreckenberger, P Bartenstein, *et al.* Positron emission tomography for staging esophageal carcinoma: Does it lead to a different therapeutic approach? *World J Surg*, **27** (2003), 1105–12.

27. J. Y. Choi, K. H. Lee, Y. M. Shim, *et al.* Improved detection of individual nodal involvement in squamous cell carcinoma of the esophagus by FDG PET. *J Nucl Med*, **41** (2000), 808–15.

28. T. Lerut, W. Coosemans, P. De Leyn, *et al.* Reflections on 3-field lymphadenectomy in carcinoma of the esophagus and gastroesophageal junction. *Hepatogastrenterology*, **46** (1999), 717–25.

29. H. L. van Westreenen, M. Westerterp, P. M. Bossuyt, *et al.* Systematic review of the staging performance of 18F-fluorodeoxyglucose positron emission tomography in esophageal cancer. *J Clin Oncol*, **22** (2004), 3805–12.

30. S. Yuan, Y. Yonghua, K. S. Cliffoerd Chao, *et al.* Additional value of PET/CT over PET in assessment of locoregional lymph nodes in thoracic esophageal squamous cell cancer. *J Nucl Med*, **47** (2006), 1255–9.

31. E. Vazquez-Sequeiros. Nodal status: number or site of nodes? How to improve accuracy? Is FNA always necessary? Junctional tumors – what's N and what's M? *Endoscopy*, **38** (2006), 54–8.

32. J. D. Luketich, D. M. Friedman, T. L. Weigel, *et al.* Evaluation of distant metastases in esophageal cancer: 100 consecutive positron emission tomography scans. *Ann Thorac Surg*, **68** (1999), 1133–7.

33. K. Kinkel, Y. Lu, M. Both, *et al.* Detection of hepatic metastases from cancers of the gastro-intestinal tract by using non-invasive imaging methods (US, CT, MR Imaging, PET): A meta-analysis. *Radiology*, **224** (2002), 748–56.

34. M. Selzner, T. F. Hany, P. Wilbrett, *et al.* Does the novel PET/CT imaging modality impact on the treatment of patients with metastatic colorectal cancer of the liver. *Ann Surg*, **240** (2004), 1027–36.

35. H. Kato, T. Miyazaki, M. Nakajima, *et al.* Comparison between whole-body positron emission tomography and bone scintigraphy in evaluating bony metastases of esophageal carcinomas. *Anticancer Res*, **25** (2005), 4439–44.

36. A. V. Taira, R. J. Herfkens, S. S. Gambhir, and A. Quon. Detection of bone metastases. Assessment of integrated FDG-PET/CT imaging. *Radiology*, **243** (2007), 204–11.

37. T. Lerut, P. Flamen, N. Ectors, *et al.* Histopathologic validation of lymph node staging with FDG-PET scan in cancer of the esophageal gastroesophageal junction: a prospective study based on primary surgery with extensive lymphadenectomy. *Ann Surg*, **232** (2000), 743–51.

38. A. W. Blackstock, M. R. Farmer, J. Lovato, *et al.* A prospective evaluation of the impact of 18-F-fluoro-deoxy-D-glucose positron emission tomography staging on survival for patients with locally advanced esophageal cancer. *Int J Radiat Oncol Biol Phys*, **64** (2006), 455–60.

39. C. P. Duong, H. Demittiou, L. Weih, *et al.* Significant clinical impact and prognostic stratification provided by FDG-PET in the staging of oesophageal cancer. *Eur J Nucl Med Mol Imaging*, **33** (2006), 759–69.

40. A. Stahl, J. Stollfus, K. Ott, *et al.* FDG PET and CT in locally advanced adenocarcinoma of the distal oesophagus. *Nuklearmedizin*, **44** (2005), 249–55.

41. [H. Jadvar, R. W. Henderson, and P. S. Conti. 2-Deoxy-2-[F-18] fluoro-D-glucose-positron emission tomography/computed tomography imaging evaluation of esophageal carcinoma.] *Mol Imaging Biol*, **8** (2006), 193–200.

42. H. L. van Westreenen, P. A. Heeren, and H. M. van Dullemen. Positron emission tomography with F-18-fluorodeoxyglucose in a combined staging strategy of esophageal cancer prevents unnecessary surgical explorations. *J Gastrointest Surg*, **9** (2005), 54–61.

43. H. L. van Westreenen, P. A. Heeren, P. L. Jager, *et al.* Pitfalls of positive findings in staging esophageal cancer with F-18-fluorodeoxyglucose positron emission tomography. *Ann of Surg Oncol*, **10** (2003), 1100–5.

44. F. Dehdashti and B. A. Siegel. Neoplasms of the esophagus and stomach. *Semin Nuclear Med*, **34** (2004), 198–208.

45. M. B. Wallace, P. J. Nietert, C. Earle, *et al.* An analysis of multiple staging management strategies for carcinoma of the esophagus: Computed tomography, endoscopic ultrasound, positron emission tomography, and thoracoscopy/laparoscopy. *Ann Thorac Surg*, **74** (2002), 1026–32.

46. A. Imdahl, M. Hentschel, M. Kleimaier, *et al.* Impact of FDG-PET for staging of oesophageal cancer. *Langenbecks Arch Surg*, **389** (2004), 283–8.

47. H. Shimada, S. Okazumi, H. Matsubara, *et al.* Impact of the number and extent of positive lymph nodes in 200 patients with thoracic esophageal squamous cell carcinoma after three-field lymph node dissection. *World J Surg*, **30** (2006), 1441–9.

48. Y. Gu, S. G. Swisher, J. A. Ajani, *et al.* The number of lymph nodes with metastasis predicts survival in patients with esophageal or esophagogastric junction adenocarcinoma who receive preoperative chemoradiation. *Cancer*, **106** (2006), 1017–25.

49. J. Y. Choi, H. J. Jang, Y. M. Shim, *et al.* 18F-FDG PET in patients with esophageal squamous cell carcinoma undergoing curative surgery: prognostic implications. *J Nucl Med*, **45** (2004), 1843–50.

50. R. J. Cerfolio and A. S. Bryant. Maximum standardized uptake values on positron emission tomography of esophageal cancer predicts stage, tumour biology, and survival. *Ann Thorac Surg*, **82** (2006), 391–5.

51. N. Rizk, R. J. Downey, T. Akhurst, *et al.* Preoperative 18-F-fluorodeoxyglucose positron emission tomography standardized uptake values predict survival after esophageal adenocarcinoma resection. *Ann Thorac Surg*, **81** (2006), 1076–81.

52. O. Vrieze, K. Haustermans, W. de Wever, *et al.* Is there a role for FDG-PET in radiotherapy planning in esophageal carcinoma? *Radiother Oncol*, **73** (2004), 269–75.

53. T. Leong, C. Everitt, K. Yuen, *et al.* A prospective study to evaluate the impact of FDG-PET on CT-based radiotherapy treatment planning for oesophageal cancer. *Radiother Oncol*, **78** (2006), 254–61.

54. L. Moureau-Zabotto, E. Touboul, D. Lerouge, *et al.* Impact of CT and 18-deoxyglucose positron emission tomography image fusion for conformal radiotherapy in esophageal carcinoma. *Int J Radiat Oncol Biol Phys*, **63** (2005), 340–5.

55. A. Konski, M. Doss, B. Milestone, *et al.* The integration of 18-fluoro-deoxy-glucose positron emission tomography and endoscopic ultrasound in the treatment-planning process for esophageal carcinoma. *Int J Radiat Oncol Biol Phys*, **61** (2005), 1123–8.

56. J. D. Urschel and H. Vasan. A meta-analysis of randomized controlled trials that compared neoadjuvant chemoradiation and surgery to surgery alone for resectable esophageal cancer. *Am J Surg*, **185** (2003), 538–43.

57. Medical Research Oesophageal Cancer Working Group. Surgical resection with or without preoperative chemotherapy in oesophageal cancer: a randomised controlled trial. *Lancet*, **359** (2002), 1727–33.

58. J. I. Geh, A. M. Crellin, and R. Glynne-Jones. Preoperative (neoadjuvant) chemoradiotherapy in oesophageal cancer. *Br J Surg*, **88** (2001), 338–56.

59. R. J. Korst, A. L. Kansler, J. L. Port, *et al.* Downstaging of T or N predicts long-term survival after preoperative chemotherapy and radical resection for esophageal carcinoma. *Ann Thorac Surg*, **82** (2006), 480–4.

60. E. A. Levine, N. R. Farmer, P. Clark, *et al.* Predictive value of 18-fluoro-deoxy-glucose-positron emission tomography (18F-FDG-PET) in the identification of responders to chemoradiation therapy for the treatment of locally advanced esophageal cancer. *Ann Surg*, **243** (2006), 472–8.

61. M. E. Juweid and B. D. Cheson. Positron-emission tomography and assessment of cancer therapy. *N Engl J Med*, **354** (2006), 496–507.

62. L. Kostakoglu and S. J. Goldsmith. PET in the assessment of therapy response in patients with carcinoma of the head and neck and of the esophagus. *J Nucl Med*, **45** (2004), 56–68.

63. L. Kostakoglu and S. J. Goldsmith. ^{18}F-FDG PET evaluation of the response to therapy for lymphoma and for breast, lung, and colorectal carcinoma. *J Nucl Med*, **44** (2003), 224–39.

64. W. A. Weber, K. Ott, K. Becker, *et al*. Prediction of response to preoperative chemotherapy in adenocarcinomas of the esophagogastric junction by metabolic imaging. *J Clin Oncol*, **19** (2001), 3058–65.

65. K. Ott, W. A. Weber, F. Lordick, *et al*. Metabolic imaging predicts response, survival, and recurrence in adenocarcinomas of the esophagogastric junction. *J Clin Oncol*, **24** (2006), 4692–8.

66. H. A. Wieder, A. J. Beer, F. Lordick, *et al*. Comparison of changes in tumour metabolic activity and tumour size during chemotherapy of adenocarcinomas of the esophagogastric junction. *J Nucl Med*, **46** (2005), 2029–34.

67. H. A. Wieder, B. L. D. M. Brucher, F. Zimmermann, *et al*. Time course of tumour metabolic activity during chemoradiotherapy of esophageal squamous cell carcinoma and response to treatment. *J Clin Oncol*, **22** (2004), 900–8.

68. C. M. Gillham, J. A. Lucey, M. Keogan, *et al*. [18]FDDG uptake during induction chemoradiation for oesophageal cancer fails to predict histomorphological tumour. *Br J Cancer*, **95** (2006), 1174–9.

69. P. Flamen, E. Van Cutsem, T. Lerut, *et al*. Positron emission tomography for assessment of the response to induction radiochemotherapy for locally advanced esophagus cancer. *Ann Oncol*, **13** (2002), 361–8.

70. B. L. Brucher, W. Weber, M. Bauer, *et al*. Neoadjuvant therapy of esophageal squamous cell carcinoma: response evaluation by positron emission tomography. *Ann Surg*, **233** (2001), 300–9.

71. M. Westerterp, H. L. van Westreenen, J. B. Reitsma, *et al*. Esophageal cancer: CT, endoscopic US and FDG PET for assessment of response to neoadjuvant therapy – Systematic review. *Radiology*, **236** (2005), 841–51.

72. A. J. Beer, H. A. Wieder, F. Lordick, *et al*. Adenocarcinomas of esophagogastric junction: multi-detector row CT to evaluate early response to neoadjuvant chemotherapy. *Radiology*, **239** (2006), 472–80.

73. S. G. Swisher, M. Maish, J. J. Erasmus, *et al*. Utility of PET, CT and EUS to identify pathologic responders in esophageal cancer. *Ann Thorac Surg*, **78** (2004), 1152–60.

74. C. P. Duong, R. J. Hicks, L. Weih, *et al*. FDG-PET status following chemoradiotherapy provides high management impact and powerful prognostic stratification in oesophageal cancer. *Eur J Nucl Med Mol Imaging*, **33** (2006), 770–8.

75. S. K. Y. Law, M. Fok, and J. Wong. Pattern of recurrence after esophageal resection for cancer: clinical implications. *Br J Surg*, **83** (1996), 107–11.

76. S. J. Lee, K. S. Lee, Y. J. Yim, *et al*. Recurrence of squamous cell carcinoma of the oesophagus after curative surgery: rates and patterns on imaging studies correlated with tumour location and pathological stage. *Clin Radiol*, **60** (2005), 547–54.

77. J. L. Raoul, E. Le Prise, B. Meunier, *et al*. Combined radiochemotherapy for postoperative recurrence of esophageal cancer. *Gut*, **37** (1995), 174–6.

78. P. Flamen, T. Lerut, E. Van Cutsem, *et al.* The utility of positron emission tomography (PET) for the diagnosis staging of recurrent esophageal cancer. *J Thorac Cardiovasc Surg,* **120** (2000), 1085–92.

79. H. Kato, T. Miyazaki, M. Nakajima, *et al.* Value of positron emission tomography in the diagnosis of recurrent esophageal carcinoma. *Br J Surg,* **91** (2004), 1004–9.

80. J. D. Zhang, J. M. Yu, H. B. Guo, *et al.* [Clinical value of positron emission tomography-CT for the diagnosis of postoperative recurrence and metastasis in the patients with oesophageal cancer] [Article in Chinese]. *Zhonhua Wei Chang Wai Ke Za Zhi,* **9** (2006), 56–8.

7

The Role of Surgery in the Management of Esophageal Cancer and Palliation of Inoperable Disease

Robert Mason

Introduction

In spite of improvements in diagnosis, staging, and treatment, the outcome for patients with esophageal cancer remains poor. Although 1-year survival has improved in recent years, there has been little change in the 5-and 10-year survival (Figure 7.1). This is because many of the patients have metastatic disease, with a large percentage having micrometastases. These have been found in the bone marrow in patients undergoing resection in 88% of cases [1].

A significant factor in the improved 1-year survival is the reduction in inhospital operative mortality (Table 7.1) [1,2,3,4]. This relates to improvement in staging, fitness testing, technique, perioperative care, and probably most importantly centralization of services in large centers (Table 7.2) [5,6,7]. In a study from the United Kingdom there was a 40% reduction in operative mortality for every 10 patient increase in a surgeon's caseload. [8]. Such large centers with dedicated teams can achieve inhospital mortality figures of less than 2% by utilizing a multidisciplinary team approach [4].

Another factor in improved short-term survival is the recognition that surgery alone is not the answer for most cases and that survival benefits can accrue by the use of preoperative neoadjuvant chemotherapy and possible chemoradiotherapy [9]. This is certainly now the practice in the United Kingdom for all cases other than early T1/2 N0 disease. Whether such treatment acts as a prolongation of disease-free interval only or improves long-term cure remains to be determined. What is evident is that preoperative chemotherapy identifies a group of patients with aggressive disease who would do very badly with surgery – "selection by oncology."

Carcinoma of the Esophagus, ed. Sheila C. Rankin. Published by Cambridge University Press. © Cambridge University Press 2008.

Table 7.1 Results of esophagectomy over time

Time period	Inhospital mortality (%)	One-year survival (%)
1960–1979[1]	29	45
1980–1988[2]	13	56
1990–2000[3]	9	63
2000–2003[4]	1.1	78

Table 7.2 Does volume of cases matter in esophageal surgery

(a) USA: Data from 1994 to 1999 (mortality corrected for coexisting conditions)

Number of cases performed/year	Observed mortality (%) ($p < 0.001$)
<2	20.3
2–4	17.8
5–7	16.2
8–19	11.4
>19	8.4

Surgeon volume more important than hospital volume [5,6].

(b) Holland [7]

Number of cases performed/year	Hospital mortality (%)
1–10	12.1
11–20	7.5
>50	4.9

Accurate preoperative staging and discussion in multidisciplinary meetings enable patients to be allocated to primary surgery for T1/2 N0 tumors, and neoadjuvant chemotherapy (possibly with radiotherapy) followed by resection, if no disease progression, for all T3 and N1 disease. Patients with M1a disease or T4 tumors involving the crura are also potential surgical candidates if significant response has been seen with neoadjuvant therapy.

The majority of patients, however, will not be suitable for surgery at any stage of their disease and require palliation of dysphagia by either intubation or recanalization.

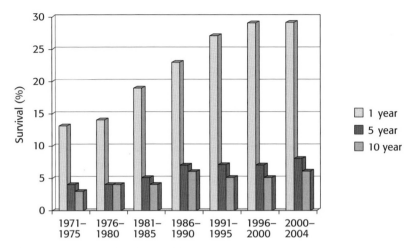

Figure 7.1 Outcomes for patients with esophageal cancer over time.

Surgery

When considering a patient for surgery, there are three fundamental principles that must be understood prior to the patient undergoing resection.

The first is that the patient must survive the procedure. This requires careful assessment of comorbidity and optimization before surgery possibly using cardiopulmonary exercise testing.

The second point is that if all goes well there must be a realistic expectation of survival in excess of 18 months. Quality-of-life studies have consistently demonstrated that patients whose survival after resection is less than 18 months never regain their preoperative quality of life [10].

The third point concerns the ability to resect all disease seen on imaging as an R2 resection leaving macroscopic disease has a very poor outcome [11]. The role of PET/CT in the demonstration of small-volume metastatic disease has had a major impact on resection rates.

If these three principles cannot be achieved, the patient is best treated by nonsurgical means.

Principles of resection

The various approaches to resection of the esophagus are listed in Table 7.3 [12,13,14,15,16,17,18]. There is no agreed single approach for the esophagus in

Table 7.3 Surgical approach and lymphadenectomy

Operation	Plus	Minus
Transhiatal (THE) [12,13]	Avoids thoracotomy Reduced morbidity Anastomosis in neck	"Not a cancer operation" Only for junctional cancer
Lewis–Tanner (LT) [14,15]	Exposure Lymphadenectomy Stapled anastomosis	Thoracotomy Poor hiatal exposure Two-stage
Three-stage [16]	Total esophageal resection Lymphadenectomy Anastomosis in neck	Thoracotomy Increased morbidity Three-stage
Left thoracoabdominal [17]	Good hiatal exposure One incision	Lower-third tumors only Costal margin problems
Minimally invasive	Reduced morbidity	"Not a cancer operation" Time

all cases, and the maxim "the approach which gives best access to the most difficult aspect of the operation" holds true. Anyone undertaking resection must be familiar with all approaches. In general for tumors at the gastroesophageal junction or lower-third esophagus (Siewert Type 1 and 2) either transhiatal esophagectomy (THE), left thoraco-abdominal, or Lewis–Tanner (LT) approach (abdomen and right chest incision) are appropriate. For middle-third tumors either an LT or a three-stage resection (abdomen, right chest incision, and anastomosis in the neck) is appropriate. Upper-third tumors are now largely treated by primary chemoradiotherapy and surgery reserved in early-stage disease when a three-stage resection with possible resection of cricopharyngeus is the operation of choice.

The recent advent of minimally invasive approaches using laparoscopy and thoracoscopy to undertake the abdominal and/or chest phases of the procedure is gaining in popularity. There is no doubt that in the hands of an expert it is possible to undertake virtually the whole operation this way [19]. The operation takes longer to perform and has a significant learning curve, and there is no evidence that intra- and postoperative complications as mentioned later are any less. There are no randomized trials comparing minimally access surgery with conventional surgery, and it is unlikely that a truly randomized trial will ever be

Table 7.4 Randomized study of operative approach: two-field Lewis–Tanner (LT) versus transhiatal esophagectomy (THE) [20]

Early postoperative complications	THE	LT
Pulmonary (%)	27	56
Cardiac (%)	16	26
Anastomotic leak (%)	14	16
Right laryngeal nerve palsy (%)	13	21
Chylothorax (%)	2	10
Intensive care stay (days)	2 days	6 days
Inhospital mortality (%)	2	4
R0 resection (%)	72	71
Number of lymph nodes	16	31
Cost (euros)	24 000	37 000

Table 7.5 Results of randomized studies of operative approach [20]: two-field Lewis–Tanner (LT) versus transhiatal esophagectomy (THE)

	THE	LT
Recurrence (%)		
Local	14	12
Distant	25	18
Both	18	19
Median overall survival (years)	1.8	2.0
Three-year survival (%)	40	40
Overall 5-year survival (%)	29	39
Cost per quality of life year gained 41 500 euros		

performed due to surgeon bias and preference. Large comparative trials comparing centers good at either laparoscopic or open surgery are possible and are awaited.

There is only one significant prospective randomized controlled trial comparing open operative approaches [20]. This study from Holland compared open THE to a two-phase LT approach with two-field lymphadenectomy (Tables 7.4 and 7.5).

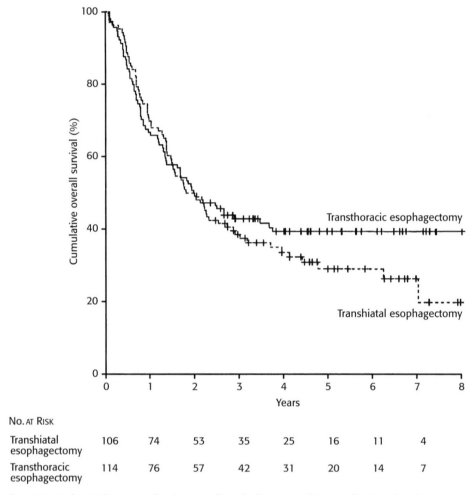

No. AT RISK

Transhiatal esophagectomy	106	74	53	35	25	16	11	4
Transthoracic esophagectomy	114	76	57	42	31	20	14	7

Figure 7.2 Kaplan–Meier curves showing overall survival among patients randomly assigned to transhiatal esophagectomy or transthoracic esophagectomy with extended en bloc lymphadenectomy. (Hulscher *et al.* Copyright 2002 Massachusetts Medical Society. All rights reserved [20]).

This demonstrated that there was no significant survival benefit (Figure 7.2) to the more radical approach that involves a thoracotomy, when compared with transhiatal resection, but the more radical approach was associated with significantly more complications. This is in agreement with data from meta-analyses (Table 7.6) [21].

Table 7.6 Meta-analysis comparing transhiatal esophagectomy (THE) and two-field Lewis–Tanner (LT) resection

	THE	LT
Number of cases	2675	2808
Morbidity (%)		
Respiratory	24	25
Cardiovascular	12.4	10.5
Chylothorax	2.1	3.4
Anastomotic leak	16	10
Stricture	28	16
Recurrent laryngeal nerve palsy	11.2	4.8
Thirty-day mortality (%)	6.3	9.5
Five-year survival (%)	24	26

Review of 62 papers published from 1986 to 1996 [21].

Lymphadenectomy

Controversy also exists as to the extent of lymphadenectomy performed at surgery. The pattern of spread for adenocarcinoma is to paraesophageal nodes and then to the left gastric and celiac nodes. In contrast, for squamous cell carcinoma isolated metastases to nodes out with the local field occurs in up to one-third of cases [22].

The standard approach whether by transhiatal or by transthorasic approach involves a one-field lymphadenectomy involving the left gastric and common hepatic nodes especially for adenocarcinoma of the lower third and esophagogastric junction. Advocates of more radical two-field lymphadenectomy removing intrathoracic nodes including subcarinal glands claim a reduction in local recurrence but no significant survival benefits [23]. There is no doubt that the more glands removed the more accurate the staging (stage migration) and a minimum of 12 glands are required to stage accurately. Those patients with more than four positive glands do have a significantly worse prognosis. The Dutch study already alluded to could show no benefit for the more radical lymphadenectomy, and there is no proven benefit for removal of the thoracic duct.

The recognition that patients with squamous carcinoma can have isolated lymph node metastases out with the local lymphatic field has lead some to advocate radical three-field lymphadenectomy involving the neck in addition to the mediastinum and abdomen. This approach is particularly popular in Japan. In the West where the majority of malignancy is adenocarcinoma, more radical three-field lymphadenectomy has no proven benefit, although in small series of highly selected patients there may be some survival benefit [24], but there is increased incidence of complications.

Replacement conduit

Having removed the esophagus, how should it be replaced? Consensus dictates that the stomach in the form of a thin gastric tube functions best and appears to have a lower failure rate from ischemia. Both right and left colonic pedicles can be used if stomach is not available. The routine use of pyloroplasty is controversial. The only randomized trials show no benefit for such a procedure in preventing stasis in the gastric tube especially if a narrow tube is used [25]. Jejunum can be used for junctional tumors but, if brought higher, usually requires a microvascular anastomosis to maintain viability. It is accepted that the preferred route for immediate reconstruction is the posterior mediastinum [26] approach used. Neck anastomoses are associated with a higher leak and stricture rate than those performed in the chest. However, death from a neck leak is extremely rare in contrast to a symptomatic leak in the chest, which can result in mortality in up to 10% of cases. The incidence of anastomotic complications does not appear to be related to technique whether staples or sutures are used. Good blood supply and lack of tension are the crucial factors.

Complications of esophageal resection

As described earlier, complications following esophagectomy occur in up to one-third of cases. Apart from generalized complications of major surgery, esophagectomy is associated with specific complications that have a significant impact on morbidity and mortality. These include chylothorax, recurrent laryngeal nerve palsy, conduit failure, and anastomotic leakage and stricture.

Chylothorax resulting from damage to the thoracic duct is usually managed conservatively with total parenteral nutrition unless loss exceeds 500 ml/day for 2 days. In this case reexploration via the right chest is required. It is best prevented by formal identification and ligation of the thoracic duct at T10 at the time of lymphadenectomy.

Recurrent laryngeal nerve injury usually involves the left nerve and occurs at the time of intrathoracic lymphadenectomy or when the esophagus is mobilized in the left neck for anastomosis following transhiatal resection. Awareness and preservation is the best prevention. Damage to one nerve produces problems with coughing and hoarseness of voice. It can be treated by injection of collagen or Teflon. Bilateral nerve injury necessitates a tracheostomy.

Major conduit failure presents within 24–48 hours as a rapid deterioration and presence of GI fluids in chest drains. Early recognition and return to theater are mandatory. The reason for failure is usually technical/ischemia and necessitates conduit removal, a cervical esophagostomy, and a feeding jejunostomy. Reconstruction can be undertaken using either left colon or supercharged jejunum either substernal or subcutaneous at a later date [27]. If the defect is a short area of necrosis on the staple line of a gastric tube and the tube as a whole is viable, local excision and suture with or without a T tube can be performed.

Radiological leaks with no clinical upset can be managed conservatively but if associated with major deterioration of the clinical picture and sepsis may require conduit resection as described. The use of removable plastic stents has been advocated but must be used with extreme caution.

Anastomotic stricture is more common with neck anastomoses and is usually due to ischemia. They invariably respond to endoscopic balloon dilatation, although this may need to be repeated and in rare instances the stricture stented – preferably with a removable plastic stent. Stenoses appearing late – in excess of 6 months postoperative – should alert the clinician to local recurrence.

Postoperative management

In the postoperative management of patients undergoing esophagectomy, controversy exists as to the wisdom of postoperative ventilation [28]. Recent studies have suggested that patients can be safely extubated on table at the end of surgery. These series all have a higher inhospital mortality than our unit where elective ventilation is the rule [4,29]. The logic for ventilation is to optimize oxygen delivery to the tissues in the crucial first 24 hours. It is likely that selective extubation when certain agreed "goals" are reached is the best answer. The lack of proper intensive care backup must not be used as an excuse for suboptimal management. It is now accepted that postoperative feeding benefits the patient and that this is best administered enterally via a feeding jejunostomy tube.

Palliation of malignant dysphagia

In spite of improvement discussed earlier, the majority of patients will not be suitable for surgery either due to advanced disease or due to comorbidity and poor fitness levels. Such patients require palliation of their symptoms particularly dysphagia. In those who are fit enough, radical therapy with chemoradiotherapy may be indicated, but most will not be able to tolerate this. In these cases relief of dysphagia can be achieved by several means. These include intubation with rigid or self-expanding tubes, or necrosis/vaporization of tumor to recanalize the esophagus.

The original methods of palliation involved the placement of rigid plastic tubes either by pulsion (Celestin) or drawing through the stricture at open surgery (Mousseau Barbin). Such tubes have been largely replaced by self-expanding metallic stents that can be placed either endoscopically or under fluoroscopic guidance. These do not require preinsertion dilatation and have lower morbidity at insertion. Several different designs are available and can be either uncovered mesh or mesh coated with plastic to reduce tumor ingrowth. These stents are not without complications that include migration, particularly in covered stents crossing the esophagogastric junction, recurrence of dysphagia, bleeding, and pain resulting from the gradual radial dilatation of the stent. This latter complication is frequently underreported and on occasions may necessitate stent removal. Migration of stents at the cardia has lead to novel designs including conical designs [30,31].

Recannalization of malignant strictures can be achieved by laser with or without photodynamic therapy, which is discussed elsewhere. It can also be achieved by argon beam photocoagulation, diathermy via a bicep, and by chemical necrosis induced by injection of absolute alcohol.

The use of palliative surgical bypass of unresectable tumors has been largely abandoned.

It appears from the literature that there is no single technique that is better in all cases. Each technique is effective in roughly two-thirds of cases and comparative studies are listed in Tables 7.7 [32,33,34,35,36] and 8 [37,38,39,40,41,42,43]. These studies usually involve small numbers of cases randomized and show little advantage for any single modality. In the largest series to date Shenfine *et al.* could not demonstrate superiority for any individual technique [44]. General consensus is that covered soft self-expanding metallic stents work best for mural and extramural disease and laser for polypoid soft intraluminal disease.

Table 7.7 Randomized trials of palliation

- Laser versus plastic tubes

No difference in relief of dysphagia or morbidity [32]

- Laser versus ethanol injection

No difference in relief of dysphagia or frequency of treatment [33]

- Laser versus brachytherapy

No difference in relief of dysphagia [34]

- Laser alone versus laser + radiotherapy (RT) or brachytherapy

The addition of RT or brachytherapy reduces the frequency of intervention, no survival benefit [35]

- Laser alone versus laser + ECF chemotherapy

ECF reduces the need for laser and possibly prolongs survival [36]

Table 7.8 Randomized trials of palliation

- Stents versus plastic tubes

Both relieve dysphagia. Stents better than plastic tubes. Less morbidity with stents [37,38,39]

- Stents versus laser

Stents better than laser at relieving dysphagia [40]

- Stents versus laser + radiotherapy

More re-stenosis, greater morbidity/mortality with laser plus radiotherapy [41]

- Stents versus thermal ablation

Thermal ablation has a survival benefit over stents. Stents cause more pain than thermal ablation [42]

- Stents versus surgical bypass

Better relief of dysphagia with stents. Mortality with surgery 25% [43]

The serious complication of perforated carcinoma or malignant tracheoesophageal fistula is best treated by stenting, although for high fistulae parallel esophageal and tracheal stents may be required (Figure 7.3) [45].

Conclusions

- The significant increase in the incidence of esophageal cancer in the West is a result of adenocarcinoma around the gastroesophageal junction.
- Patients with T3 and/or N1 disease benefit from multimodal therapy.

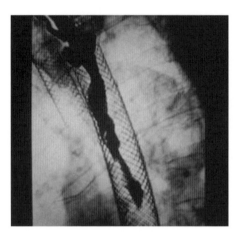

Figure 7.3 Parallel covered stents in the trachea and esophagus for a high malignant tracheoesophageal fistula.

- Prior to consideration of surgery, full assessment of fitness and staging must be undertaken.
- Centralization of services improves outcome of surgery with regard to morbidity and mortality.
- No single operative approach or the extent of lymphadenectomy has been shown to be superior in the West, although adequate lymphadenectomy should be performed to enable correct staging.
- For palliation, all techniques appear to be equally effective.
- For complications such as fistula or perforation, covered self-expanding metallic stents are the treatment of choice.

REFERENCES

1. G. C. O'Sullivan, D. Sheehan, A. Clarke, *et al.* Micrometastases in esophagogastric cancer: high detection rate in resected rib segments. *Gastroenterology*, **116** (1999), 543–8.
2. J. M. Muller, H. Erasmi, M. Stelzner, U. Zieren, and H. Pichmaier. Surgical therapy of oesophageal carcinoma. *Br J Surg*, **77** (1990), 845–57.
3. G. G. Jamieson, G. Mathew, R. Ludemann, *et al.* Postoperative mortality following oesophagectomy and problems in reporting its rate. *Br J Surg*, **91** (2004), 943–7.
4. M. J. Forshaw, J. A. Gossage, J. Stephens, *et al.* Centralisation of oesophagogastric cancer services: can specialist units deliver? *Ann R Coll Surg Engl*, **88**:6 (2006), 566–70.
5. J. D. Birkmeyer, A. E. Siewers, E. V. A. Finlayson, *et al.* Hospital volume and surgical mortality in the United States. *N Engl J Med*, **346** (2002), 1128–37.

6. J. D. Birkmeyer, T. A. Stukel, A. E. Siewers, *et al*. Surgeon volume and operative mortality in the United States. *N Engl J Med*, **349** (2003), 2117–27.

7. J. J. B. van Lanschot, J. B. F. Hulscher, C. J. Buskens, *et al*. Hospital volume and hospital mortality for esophagectomy. *Cancer*, **91** (2001), 1574–8.

8. M. O. Bachmann, D. Alderson, D. Edwards, *et al*. Cohort study in South and West England of the influence of specialization on the management and outcome of patients with oesophageal and gastric cancers. *Br J Surg*, **89** (2002), 914–22.

9. Medical Research Council Oesophageal Cancer Working Group. Surgical resection with or without preoperative chemotherapy in oesophageal cancer: a randomised controlled trial. *Lancet*, **359**:9319 (2002), 1727–33.

10. J. M. Blazeby, M. H. Williams, S. T. Brookes, *et al*. Quality of life measurement in patients with oesophageal cancer. *Gut*, **37**:4 (1995), 505–8.

11. T. Lerut, P. W. de Leyn, W. Coosemans *et al*. Surgical strategies in esophageal carcinoma with emphasis on radical lymphadenectomy. *Ann Surg*, **216**:5 (1992), 583–90.

12. M. B. Orringer. Transhiatal esophagectomy without thoracotomy for carcinoma of the thoracic esophagus. *Ann Surg*, **200** (1984), 282–8.

13. D. Alderson, S. P. Courtney, and R. H. Kennedy. Radical transhiatal oesophagectomy under direct vision. *Br J Surg*, **81** (1994), 404–7.

14. H. Akiyama, M. Tsurumaru, H. Udagawa, and Y. Kajiyama. Radical lymph node dissection for cancer of the thoracic esophagus. *Ann Surg*, **220** (1994), 364–73.

15. D. N. Sutton, J. Wayman, and S. M. Griffin. Learning curve for oesophageal cancer surgery *Br J Surg*, **85** (1998), 1399–402.

16. D. B. Skinner. En bloc resection for neoplasms of the esophagus and cardia. *J Thorac Cardiovasc Surg*, **85** (1983), 59–71.

17. M. J. Forshaw, J. A. Gossage, J. Ockrim, S. W. Atkinson, and R. C. Mason. Left thoracoabdominal esophagogastrectomy: still a valid operation for carcinoma of the distal esophagus and esophagogastric junction. *Dis Esophagus*, **19** (2006), 340–5.

18. J. D. Luketich, P. R. Schauer, N. A. Christie, *et al*. Minimally invasive esophagectomy. *Ann Thorac Surg*, **70** (2000), 906–11.

19. C. Bizekis, M. S. Kent, J. Luketich, *et al*. Initial experience with minimally invasive Ivor Lewis esophagectomy. *Ann Thorac Surg*, **82**:2 (2006), 402–6.

20. J. B. Hulscher, J. W. van Sandick, A. G. de Boer, *et al*. Extended transthoracic resection compared with limited transhiatal resection for adenocarcinoma of the esophagus. *N Engl J Med*, **347** (2002), 1662–9. Comment in *N Engl J Med*, 347 (2002), 1705–9.

21. R. Rindani, C. J. Martin, and M. R. Cox. Transhiatal versus Ivor–Lewis oesophagectomy: is there a difference? *Aust and N Z Surg*, **69** (1999), 187–94.

22. J. Wayman, M. K. Bennett, S. A. Raimes, *et al*. The pattern of recurrence of adenocarcinoma of the oesophago-gastric junction. *Br J Cancer*, **86**:8 (2002), 1223–9.

23. S. M. Dresner and S. M. Griffin. Pattern of recurrence following radical oesophagectomy with two-field lymphadenectomy. *Br J Surg*, **87**:10 (2000), 1426–33.

24. T. Lerut, T. Nafteux, J. Moons, *et al.* Three-field lymphadenectomy for carcinoma of the esophagus and gastroesophageal junction in 174 R0 resections: impact on staging, disease-free survival, and outcome – a plea for adaptation of TNM classification in upper-half esophageal carcinoma. *Ann Surg*, **240**:6 (2004), 962–72.

25. H. C. Cheung, K. F. Siu, and J. Wong. Is pyloroplasty necessary in esophageal replacement by stomach? A prospective, randomized controlled trial. *Surgery*, **102** (1987), 19–24.

26. A. C. Wong, S. Law, and J. Wong. Influence of the route of reconstruction on morbidity, mortality and local recurrence after esophagectomy for cancer. *Dig Surg*, **20** (2003), 209–14.

27. H. M. P. Dowson, D. Strauss, R. Ng, and R. Mason. The acute management and surgical reconstruction following failed esophagectomy in malignant disease of the esophagus. *Dis Esophagus*, **20** (2007), 135–40.

28. M. T. Caldwell, P. G. Murphy, R. Page, T. N. Walsh, and T. P. Hennessy. Timing of extubation after oesophagectomy. *Br J Surg*, **80** (1993), 1537–9.

29. S. A. Robertson, R. J. Skipworth, D. L. Clarke, *et al.* Ventilatory and intensive care requirements following oesophageal resection. *Ann R Coll Surg Engl*, **88** (2006), 354–7.

30. R. C. Mason. Palliation of malignant dysphagia: an alternative to surgery. *Ann R Coll Surg Engl*, **78**:5 (1996), 457–62.

31. A. Adam, R. Morgan, J. Ellul, and R. C. Mason. A new design of the esophageal Wallstent endoprosthesis resistant to distal migration. *AJR Am J Roentgenol*, **170**:6 (1998), 1477–81.

32. D. Alderson and P. D. Wright. Laser recanalization versus endoscopic intubation in the palliation of malignant dysphagia. *Br J Surg*, **77** (1990), 1151–3.

33. A. Carazzone, L. Bonavina, A. Segalin, C. Ceriani, and A. Peracchia. Endoscopic palliation of oesophageal cancer: results of a prospective comparison of Nd:YAG laser and ethanol injection. *Eur J Surg*, **165** (1999), 351–6.

34. D. E. Low and K. M. Pagliero. Prospective randomized clinical trial comparing brachytherapy and laser photoablation for palliation of esophageal cancer. *J Thorac Cardiovasc Surg*, **104** (1992), 173–8.

35. I. R. Sargeant, J. S. Tobias, G. Blackman, *et al.* Radiotherapy enhances laser palliation of malignant dysphagia: a randomised study. *Gut*, **40** (1997), 362–9.

36. M. S. Highley, F. X. Parnis, G. A. Trotter, *et al.* Combination chemotherapy with epirubicin, cisplatin and 5-fluorouracil for the palliation of advanced gastric and oesophageal adenocarcinoma. *Br J Surg*, **81**:12 (1994), 1763–5.

37. K. Knyrim, H. J. Wagner, N. Bethge, M. Keymling, and N. Vakil. A controlled trial of an expansile metal stent for palliation of esophageal obstruction due to inoperable cancer. *N Engl J Med*, **329** (1993), 1302–7.

38. G. D. De Palma, E. di Matteo, G. Romano, *et al.* Plastic prosthesis versus expandable metal stents for palliation of inoperable esophageal thoracic carcinoma: a controlled prospective study. *Gastrointest Endosc*, **43** (1996), 478–82.

39. C. Sanyika, P. Corr, and A. Haffejee. Palliative treatment of oesophageal carcinoma – efficacy of plastic versus self-expandable stents. *S Afr Med J*, **89** (1999), 640–3.

40. A. Adam, J. Ellul, A. F. Watkinson, *et al.* Palliation of inoperable esophageal carcinoma: a prospective randomized trial of laser therapy and stent placement. *Radiology,* **202** (1997), 344–8.

41. A. Konigsrainer, B. Riedmann, A. de Vries, *et al.* Expandable metal stents versus laser combined with radiotherapy for palliation of unresectable esophageal cancer: a prospective randomized trial. *Hepatogastroenterology,* **47**:33 (2000), 724–7.

42. H. J. Dallal, G. D. Smith, D. C. Grieve, *et al.* A randomized trial of thermal ablative therapy versus expandable metal stents in the palliative treatment of patients with esophageal carcinoma. *Gastrointest Endosc,* **54** (2001), 549–57.

43. R. Cantero, A. J. Torres, F. Hernando, *et al.* Palliative treatment of esophageal cancer: self-expanding metal stents versus Postlethwait technique. *Hepatogastroenterology,* **46** (1999), 971–6.

44. J. Shenfine, P. McNamee, N. Steen, J. Bond, and S. M. Griffin. A pragmatic randomised controlled trial of the cost-effectiveness of palliative therapies for patients with inoperable oesophageal cancer. *Health Technol Assess,* **9**:5 (2005), iii, 1–121.

45. J. P. M. Ellul, R. Morgan, D. Gold, *et al.* Parallel self-expanding covered metal stents in the trachea and oesophagus for the palliation of complex high tracheo-oesophageal fistula. *Br J Surg,* **83**:12 (1996), 1767–8.

8

Chemotherapy and Radiotherapy in Esophageal Cancer

Peter Harper and David Landau

Introduction

Over 7600 cases of esophageal cancer are diagnosed in the United Kingdom every year. The overall survival is about 8%, and whilst there has been some improvement over time, this has not been dramatic and appears to date back to the mid 1980s (Figure 8.1) [1]. To improve these figures significantly will require prevention, earlier diagnosis, and more effective systemic therapies.

Development of chemotherapy

A UK multicenter trial, published in 1997, established epirubicin, cisplatin, and infusional 5-fluorouracil (5-FU; ECF) as the combination of choice in the UK and Europe [2]. In this study 256 patients were randomly assigned to the then standard FAMTX regime (5-fluorouracil, doxorubicin, and methotrexate) or to ECF. About 51 patients had esophageal, 60 esophagogastric, and 145 gastric cancer. The overall response rate was 45% with ECF and 21% with FAMTX ($p = 0.0002$), the median survival was 8.9 versus 5.7 months with FAMTX and, at 1 year, 36 versus 21% of the patients were alive.

With improvements in chemotherapy supportive medication, for example, the introduction of HT-3 antagonists for anti-emetic cover, cisplatin-based chemotherapy has become the treatment of choice for the majority of patients requiring chemotherapy.

Recent developments in drug therapy have increased the options for trials of systemic therapy. None has yet been proven to improve on ECF in terms of efficacy,

Carcinoma of the Esophagus, ed. Sheila C. Rankin. Published by Cambridge University Press. © Cambridge University Press 2008.

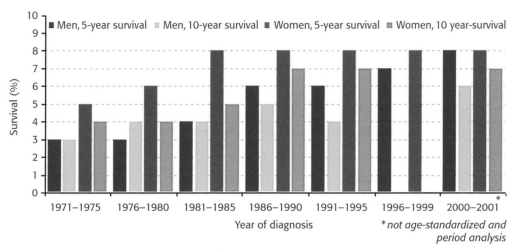

Figure 8.1 Five- and ten-year relative age-standardized survival for esophageal cancer patients aged 15–99, England and Wales, 1971–2001. (CRUK 2004 with permission [1].)

although recent trials have shown at least equivalent activity with reduced toxicity with some new agents.

Development of radiotherapy

For early disease, the RTOG 85-01 trial showed clearly that lower dose radiotherapy combined with chemotherapy was a more effective treatment than the higher dose radiotherapy alone and this is now standard treatment [3,4]. Developments in radiotherapy technology in general have led to improved target definition for esophageal irradiation as well as improved treatment delivery. The next anticipated step forward is the use of targeted radiosensitizing agents that will hopefully further widen the therapeutic window.

No definitive randomized study has been published comparing surgery with chemoradiotherapy as the local modality of treatment. There remain therefore a significant number of patients for whom either surgery or chemoradiation might be indicated. Which treatment is chosen will often have more to do with local biases and available skills than with the evidence base.

In each section of this chapter, there is a review of evidence behind current best practice, current controversies, and promising areas of research. All members of the multidisciplinary team should have knowledge of the evidence that drives the decision-making process.

Radical treatment

Neoadjuvant chemotherapy

The aim of using chemotherapy prior to surgery is twofold: first, to try and shrink the tumor prior to resection and so achieve higher complete resection rates, and second, to treat any potentially eradicable microscopic metastases as early as possible, in order to improve overall survival.

Current best practice

In 2002 Urschel *et al.* performed a meta-analysis of 11 randomized controlled trials of neoadjuvant chemotherapy, which included a total of 1976 patients [5]. A clinical response to chemotherapy was observed in 31% of patients, and 5% had a complete pathological response. Compared with surgery alone, neoadjuvant chemotherapy and surgery was associated with a lower rate of esophageal resection overall but a higher rate of complete resection. Chemotherapy did not increase treatment-related mortality, but no survival benefit was demonstrated. The largest single trial in the 2002 meta-analysis was that of Kelsen *et al.* [6], in which 440 patients were randomly allocated to receive either two cycles of the CF (cisplatin + 5-FU) regime or surgery only.

The MRC OE-02 (2002) trial randomized 802 previously untreated patients with resectable esophageal cancer of any cell type to either two cycles of preoperative CF or resection alone [7]. Resection was microscopically complete in 233 (60%) of 390 assessable chemotherapy patients and 215 (54%) of 397 surgery-only patients ($p < 0.0001$). Overall survival was better in the chemotherapy group (hazard ratio 0.79; 95% CI 0.67–0.93; $p = 0.004$). Median survival was 16.8 months in the chemotherapy group versus 13.3 months for surgery alone and 2-year survival rates were 43 and 34%, respectively (Figure 8.2). A repeat meta-analysis including the MRC trial showed a significant 4.4% improvement in 2-year survival [8]. There was no significant difference in the results between adenocarcinoma and squamous cell carcinoma.

Neoadjuvant chemotherapy is now standard treatment as a result of these trials. In general, patients with T3 disease or greater and those with clinically positive nodes are selected for preoperative chemotherapy.

Current controversies

Positron emission tomography (PET) offers the potential to predict at an early stage which patients are responding to therapy and which not. This would allow

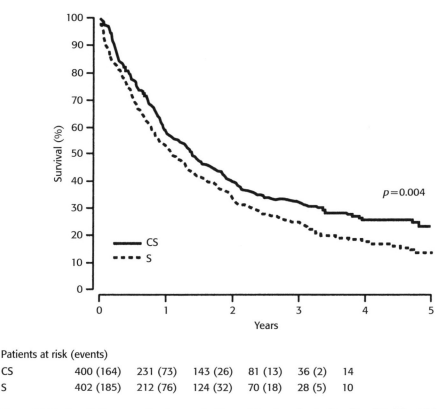

Patients at risk (events)

CS	400 (164)	231 (73)	143 (26)	81 (13)	36 (2)	14
S	402 (185)	212 (76)	124 (32)	70 (18)	28 (5)	10

Figure 8.2 Kaplan–Meier curve showing survival from date of randomization. (Reprinted from [7], with permission from Elsevier.)

intensification of therapy in responders and early abandonment to surgery in nonresponders [9,10]. However, no definitive trial has yet been completed on this question.

Promising areas of research

The current OE-05, CRUK-sponsored study in the UK compares two different chemotherapy schedules in the neoadjuvant setting: two cycles of CF versus four cycles of epirubicin, cisplatin, and capecitabine (ECX), which has been shown in the REAL 2 trial to be effective in advanced disease (see section on palliative chemotherapy).

Recent studies in lung cancer have demonstrated that platinum sensitivity might be predicted on histological specimens [11]. These, and other similar investigations, have clear applications to esophageal cancer as well as many other tumor types.

Neoadjuvant chemoradiation

The rationale for this is similar to neoadjuvant chemotherapy but recognizes the fact that a high proportion of patients fail locoregionally after surgery. Chemoradiotherapy is aimed at intensifying the locoregional therapy whilst not compromising on systemic treatment.

Current best practice

There is no routine role for trimodality therapy. It is likely that there are patients who will benefit from this approach, although their selection is not straightforward.

Current controversies

As this whole area is controversial, it is appropriate to review the available evidence in this section. Two papers have presented meta-analyses on the subject, using different criteria for selection of randomized studies that compared neoadjuvant chemoradiation with surgery alone and using different criteria for their analysis.

Kaklamanos *et al.* combined five trials totaling 669 patients and used absolute differences in survival as the main endpoint [8]. They found a benefit of 6.4% (95% CI 1.2–14.0) in 2-year survival for patients receiving neoadjuvant chemoradiotherapy, with no evidence of heterogeneity between trials. Surgical mortality was increased by 3.4% (95% CI 0.1–7.3). Urschel *et al.* identified nine studies totaling 1116 patients and used odds ratio figures to investigate the combined data [12]. Having pointed out the significant heterogeneity of the clinical schedules, they report a combined improvement in both locoregional recurrence (OR 0.38, 95% CI 0.23–0.63; $p = 0.0002$) and R0 resection rates (OR 0.53, 95% CI 0.33–0.84; $p = 0.007$). This translated into a 2-year survival advantage (OR 0.66, 95% CI 0.47–0.92; $p = 0.016$). They too found evidence of increased surgical mortality (OR 1.72, 95% CI 0.96–3.07; $p = 0.07$).

Combined, these two meta-analyses provide some basis for selective trimodality and a very good background for a definitive randomized trial to compare different neoadjuvant approaches. To date no comparison between neoadjuvant chemotherapy and neoadjuvant chemoradiation is available.

Definitive chemoradiation

Current best practice

The RTOG 85-10 trial compared the outcome of 121 patients randomly allocated to either 64 Gy in 32 fractions radiotherapy alone or 50 Gy in 25 fractions plus four cycles of CF, of which the first two were concomitant with radiation [3,4]. Median survival in the combined therapy group was 14 months compared to 9.3 months in the radiotherapy only group, and 5-year survival in the combined therapy group was 27 versus 0%. The trial was stopped early after an interim analysis.

A subsequent Intergroup trial compared the same combination to one with an increased dose of radiotherapy, 64 Gy in 32 fractions [13]. No further advantage accrued from the more intensive treatment.

Radiotherapy planning should be performed with a CT-planned, 3D, conformal therapy technique. The safety of the treatment is measured by use of dose–volume histograms that describe the distribution of radiation in normal tissues. Particular care must be taken to avoid overtreatment of the lungs. More recently, our attention has been drawn to cardiac exposure [14,15]. Unfortunately, long-term outcomes need to improve significantly before this becomes a problem for the majority of patients.

Current controversies

The role of PET is always a good topic for controversy, and this is certainly true for radiotherapy planning. Two studies have investigated the impact of PET on target definition for radiotherapy planning and confirmed that it may well have a useful role (Figure 8.3) [16,17].

Intensity-modulated radiotherapy (IMRT) is a delivery technique, based on high-technology planning algorithms, that produces highly conformal treatment plans. This means that the shape of the high-dose radiotherapy region more closely matches the exact shape of the target. Studies have shown that this is likely to decrease the exposure of normal lung tissue [18,19]. Since radiation pneumonitis is not a dose-limiting toxicity, however, and given that there seems to be no benefit to dose escalation, it remains to be seen what role IMRT will have in esophageal cancer.

Promising areas of research

As in all areas of radiotherapy, the potential of combinations with relatively nontoxic targeted agents is being investigated. The SCOPE 1 trial, being set up

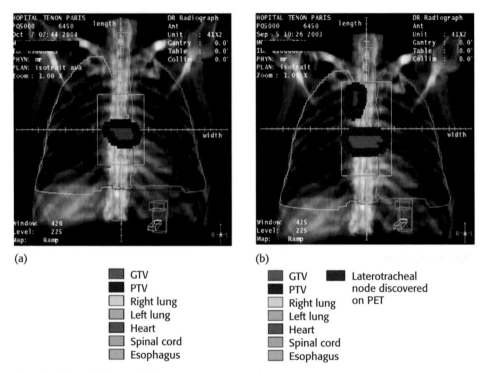

Figure 8.3 Impact of computed tomography (CT) and ^{18}F-fluoro-deoxy-D-glucose-positron emission tomography (FDG-PET) image fusion for delineation of gross tumor volume (GTV). (a) Virtual simulation with CT alone. (b) Virtual simulation with CT and FDG image fusion. Orange, GTV; purple, planning target volume (PTV); yellow, right lung; blue, left lung; pink, heart; green, spinal cord; dark yellow, esophagus; violet, lateral tracheal node discovered on PET. (Reprinted from [16], with permission from Elsevier.)

by the CRUK Upper GI Group, will investigate the addition of bevacizumab, a vascular-targeted agent, to the standard radical chemoradiation schedule.

Adjuvant chemotherapy or chemoradiation

This is treatment administered following radical surgery to reduce the risk of relapse.

Current best practice

There are no randomized data to support these treatments. Their use is limited to patients who have either been understaged preoperatively and then found to be node-positive or to have positive radial margins or to exceptional patients who were not fit for preoperative therapy but are fit for postoperative.

One study of 59 patients reported improved results compared to historical controls when treating with cisplatin and paclitaxel after surgery [20]. In general, patients are given the benefit of the doubt that they might reap similar benefits to preoperative patients, although practices vary.

Adjuvant chemoradiation is usually reserved for patients with positive radial margins. What constitutes a positive radial margin is not clear, although less than 1 mm may be used with some justification [21]. Data from the limited studies available are conflicting and in no way provide definitive support for adjuvant chemoradiation [22,23,24].

Palliative treatment

Chemotherapy

This is chemotherapy given without curative intent. The label "palliative" is misleading, as it implies that the main purpose of the treatment is to improve symptoms. The inference that symptom-free patients should therefore not receive chemotherapy is by no means true. In the modern world of multicenter oncology trials, no new regimen can be introduced into the clinic purely on the basis that it palliates symptoms; there must be a survival advantage too. There is usually far more to be gained with chemotherapy, even in a noncurative setting, than with simple palliation.

First line

Current best practice

As described in the introduction to this chapter, ECF chemotherapy has been the standard regime in use since the mid 1990s. More recently, the REAL 2 trial investigated the switch of cisplatin to the less toxic oxaliplatin and of continuous intravenous infusional 5-FU to oral capecitabine [25,26]. Again, patients with esophageal, GOJ, and gastric cancers were included. A total of 964 patients were recruited into a four-arm trial. Overall, survival with the new drugs was not worse than with the older regime (it may even have been slightly better), whilst response rates seemed to be generally better with the new regimes. Toxicities were swapped rather predictably with less neutropenia and renal toxicity with oxaliplatin but more neurotoxicity. Likewise, capecitabine resulted in more lethargy and hand–foot syndrome but allowed the omission of the indwelling venous catheter.

Other smaller studies have also recently shown a similar trend toward improved efficacy and reduced toxicity with oxaliplatin and capecitabine [27,28]. There is now, therefore, the option to design the drug combination according to individual patient's needs.

Current controversies
The standard regime in the USA has been CF, i.e., ECF without the epirubicin but with a higher dose of cisplatin. This is based on a small study of less than 100 patients that used single agent as a comparator [29]. The response rate was 35% (versus 19% with cisplatin alone) and the median survival 33 weeks, compared to 40% and 10 months with ECF (comparing across trials). In the most recently reported International CF trial (like REAL 2, switching 5-FU to capecitabine), the response rate was 29% and the median survival 9.3 months [27]. It is not possible to say whether ECF or CF is the better regime without a direct comparison.

The majority of trials have recruited patients separately into protocols for gastric and GOJ and for esophageal cancers. It remains to be seen whether there is a meaningful distinction between the two groups in the context of advanced disease.

Promising areas of research
In order to improve results from systemic therapy, new drugs have been investigated. These include taxotere [30] and irinotecan [31]. The most exciting developments are likely to come with the introduction of new targeted agents. As an example, a recent US multicenter phase II trial including 47 patients with GOJ or gastric cancers investigated a schedule of cisplatin, irinotecan, and bevacizumab (a new vascular-targeted agent). They showed a promising response rate of 65% and median survival of 12.3 months [32].

Second line

Current best practice
No randomized trials have been performed in this setting. Promising regimes include cisplatin and taxotere and irinotecan plus 5-FU [33,34].

Radiotherapy

Local palliation can be achieved with short courses of radiotherapy. Dysphagia can be managed with either radiotherapy or stent insertion. Radiotherapy is very useful for bleeding lesions and painful metastases.

Conclusion

This chapter is a summary of the current oncological practice in esophageal cancer. Armed with this knowledge, each member of the multidisciplinary team should be able to gain significant benefit from the review meetings.

REFERENCES

1. Cancer Research UK (CRUK). Oesophageal Cancer survival statistics. http://info.cancerresearch-uk.org/cancerstats/types/oesophagus/survival/ (2004).

2. A. Webb, D. Cunningham, J. H. Scarffe, *et al.* Randomized trial comparing epirubicin, cisplatin, and fluorouracil versus fluorouracil, doxorubicin, and methotrexate in advanced esophagogastric cancer. *J Clin Oncol*, **15** (1997), 261–7.

3. A. Herskovic, K. Martz, M. al-Sarraf, *et al.* Combined chemotherapy and radiotherapy compared with radiotherapy alone in patients with cancer of the esophagus. *N Engl J Med*, **326** (1992), 1593–8.

4. J. S. Cooper, M. D. Guo, A. Herskovic, *et al.* Chemoradiotherapy of locally advanced esophageal cancer: long-term follow-up of a prospective randomized trial (RTOG 85–01). Radiation Therapy Oncology Group. *JAMA*, **281** (1999), 1623–7.

5. J. D. Urschel, H. Vasan, and C. J. Blewett. A meta-analysis of randomized controlled trials that compared neoadjuvant chemotherapy and surgery to surgery alone for resectable esophageal cancer. *Am J Surg*, **183** (2002), 274–9.

6. D. P. Kelsen, R. Ginsberg, T. F. Parak, *et al.* Chemotherapy followed by surgery compared with surgery alone for localized esophageal cancer. *N Engl J Med*, **339** (1998), 1979–84.

7. Medical Research Council (MRC). Surgical resection with or without preoperative chemotherapy in oesophageal cancer: a randomised controlled trial. *Lancet*, **359**:9319 (2002), 1727–33.

8. I. G. Kaklamanos, G. R. Walker, K. Ferry, *et al.* Neoadjuvant treatment for resectable cancer of the esophagus and the gastroesophageal junction: a meta-analysis of randomized clinical trials. *Ann Surg Oncol*, **10** (2003), 754–61.

9. M. J. Forshaw, J. A. Gossage, and R. C. Mason. Neoadjuvant chemotherapy for oesophageal cancer: the need for accurate response prediction and evaluation. *Surgeon*, **3** (2005), 373–82, 422.

10. R. F. Munden, H. A. Macapinlac, J. J. Erasmus, *et al.* Esophageal cancer: the role of integrated CT-PET in initial staging and response assessment after preoperative therapy. *J Thorac Imaging*, **21** (2006), 137–45.

11. K. A. Olaussen, A. Dunant, P. Fouret, *et al.* DNA repair by ERCC1 in non-small-cell lung cancer and cisplatin-based adjuvant chemotherapy. *N Engl J Med*, **355** (2006), 983–91.

12. J. D. Urschel and H. Vasan. A meta-analysis of randomized controlled trials that compared neoadjuvant chemoradiation and surgery to surgery alone for resectable esophageal cancer. *Am J Surg*, **185** (2003), 538–43.

13. B. D. Minsky, T. F. Pajak, R. J. Ginsberg, *et al.* INT 0123 (Radiation Therapy Oncology Group 94–05) phase III trial of combined-modality therapy for esophageal cancer: high-dose versus standard-dose radiation therapy. *J Clin Oncol*, **20** (2002), 1167–74.

14. M. Cominos, M. A. Mosleh-Shirazi, D. Tait, *et al.* Quantification and reduction of cardiac dose in radical radiotherapy for oesophageal cancer. *Br J Radiol*, **78** (2005), 1069–74.

15. A. M. Gaya and R. F. Ashford. Cardiac complications of radiation therapy. *Clin Oncol*, **17** (2005), 153–9.

16. L. Moureau-Zabotto, E. Touboul, D. Lerouge, *et al.* Impact of CT and ^{18}F-deoxyglucose positron emission tomography image fusion for conformal radiotherapy in esophageal carcinoma. *Int J Radiat Oncol Biol Phys*, **63** (2005), 340–5.

17. T. Leong, C. Everitt, K. Yuen, *et al.* A prospective study to evaluate the impact of FDG-PET on CT-based radiotherapy treatment planning for oesophageal cancer. *Radiother Oncol*, **78** (2006), 254–61.

18. C. M. Nutting, J. L. Bedford, V. P. Cosgrove, *et al.* A comparison of conformal and intensity-modulated techniques for oesophageal radiotherapy. *Radiother Oncol*, **61** (2001), 157–63.

19. A. Chandra, T. M. Guerrero, H. H. Lui, *et al.* Feasibility of using intensity-modulated radiotherapy to improve lung sparing in treatment planning for distal esophageal cancer. *Radiother Oncol*, **77** (2005), 247–53.

20. M. Armanios, R. Xu, A. A. Forastiere, *et al.* Adjuvant chemotherapy for resected adenocarcinoma of the esophagus, gastro-esophageal junction, and cardia: phase II trial (E8296) of the Eastern Cooperative Oncology Group. *J Clin Oncol*, **22** (2004), 4495–9.

21. S. P. Dexter, H. Sue-Ling, M. J. McMahon, *et al.* Circumferential resection margin involvement: an independent predictor of survival following surgery for oesophageal cancer. *Gut*, **48** (2001), 667–70.

22. E. L. Bedard, R. I. Inculet, R. A. Malthaner, *et al.* The role of surgery and postoperative chemoradiation therapy in patients with lymph node positive esophageal carcinoma. *Cancer*, **91** (2001), 2423–30.

23. T. W. Rice, D. J. Adelstein, M. A. Chidel, *et al.* Benefit of postoperative adjuvant chemoradiotherapy in locoregionally advanced esophageal carcinoma. *J Thorac Cardiovasc Surg*, **126** (2003), 1590–6.

24. M. Tachibana, H. Yoshimura, S. Kinugasa, *et al.* Postoperative chemotherapy vs chemoradiotherapy for thoracic esophageal cancer: a prospective randomized clinical trial. *Eur J Surg Oncol*, **29** (2003), 580–7.

25. K. Sumpter, C. Harper-Wynne, D. Cunningham, *et al.* Report of two protocol planned interim analyses in a randomised multicentre phase III study comparing capecitabine with fluorouracil and oxaliplatin with cisplatin in patients with advanced oesophagogastric cancer receiving ECF. *Br J Cancer*, **92** (2005), 1976–83.

26. D. Cunningham, S. Rao, N. Starling, *et al.* Randomised multicentre phase III study comparing capecitabine with fluorouracil and oxaliplatin with cisplatin in patients with advanced oesophagogastric (OG) cancer: The REAL 2 trial. *J Clin Oncol*, **24** (2006), LBA4017.

27. S. Al-Batran, J. Hartmann, S. Probst, *et al*. A randomized phase III trial in patients with advanced adenocarcinoma of the stomach receiving first-line chemotherapy with fluorouracil, leucovorin and oxaliplatin (FLO) versus fluorouracil, leucovorin and cisplatin (FLP). *J Clin Oncol*, **24** (2006), LBA4016.

28. Y. Kang, W. K. Kang, D. B. Shin, *et al*. Randomized phase III trial of capecitabine/cisplatin (XP) vs. continuous infusion of 5-FU/cisplatin (FP) as first-line therapy in patients (pts) with advanced gastric cancer (AGC): efficacy and safety results. *J Clin Oncol*, **24** (2006), LBA4017.

29. H. Bleiberg, T. Conroy, B. Paillot, *et al*. Randomised phase II study of cisplatin and 5-fluorouracil (5-FU) versus cisplatin alone in advanced squamous cell oesophageal cancer. *Eur J Cancer*, **33** (1997), 1216–20.

30. J. A. Ajani, M. B. Fodor, S. A. Tjulandin, *et al*. Phase II multi-institutional randomized trial of docetaxel plus cisplatin with or without fluorouracil in patients with untreated, advanced gastric, or gastroesophageal adenocarcinoma. *J Clin Oncol*, **23** (2005), 5660–7.

31. M. E. Burge, D. Smith, C. Topham, *et al*. A phase I and II study of 2-weekly irinotecan with capecitabine in advanced gastroesophageal adenocarcinoma. *Br J Cancer*, **94** (2006), 1281–6.

32. M. A. Shah, R. K. Ramanathan, D. H. Ilson, *et al*. Multicenter phase II study of irinotecan, cisplatin, and bevacizumab in patients with metastatic gastric or gastroesophageal junction adenocarcinoma. *J Clin Oncol*, **24** (2006), 5201–6.

33. S. Lorenzen, J. Duyster, C. Lersch, *et al*. Capecitabine plus docetaxel every 3 weeks in first- and second-line metastatic oesophageal cancer: final results of a phase II trial. *Br J Cancer*, **92** (2005), 2129–33.

34. L. Assersohn, G. Brown, D. Cunningham, *et al*. Phase II study of irinotecan and 5-fluorouracil/ leucovorin in patients with primary refractory or relapsed advanced oesophageal and gastric carcinoma. *Ann Oncol*, **15** (2004), 64–9.

9

Role of Stents in the Management of Esophageal Cancer

Tarun Sabharwal and Andreas Adam

Introduction

Esophageal cancer is the sixth leading cause of death from malignant disease worldwide [1,2]. Patients may have no symptoms until the diameter of the esophageal lumen has been reduced by 50%, resulting in late presentation and poor prognosis [3]. Esophageal neoplasms are associated with a poor outcome, with an overall 5-year survival rate of less than 10%. Fewer than 50% of patients are suitable for resection at presentation, and palliation is the best option for those with irresectable lesions [3,4].

Esophageal stents for palliation

The aims of palliative treatment are maintenance of oral intake, minimizing hospital stay, relief of pain, elimination of reflux and regurgitation, and prevention of aspiration [3,5,6]. Current methods of palliation include thermal ablation [7,8,9], photodynamic therapy [10,11,12], radiotherapy [13], chemotherapy [14,15], chemical injection therapy [16,17,18], argon beam or bipolar electrocoagulation therapy [19], enteral feeding (nasogastric tube/percutaneous endoscopic gastrostomy) [20,21,22], and intubation with self-expanding metal stents (SEMS) or semirigid prosthetic tubes [5,6,23,24,25,26].

Endoluminal esophageal prostheses have been in use for over a century. A variety of tubes inserted using pulsion or traction have been described. Leroy d'Etiolles made the earliest device in 1845 of decalcified ivory, followed by Charters J. Symonds who introduced the first metal esophageal prosthesis in 1885 [27]. Esophageal stenting using SEMS is the commonest modern means of palliation and is associated with high success rates and relatively few complications.

Carcinoma of the Esophagus, ed. Sheila C. Rankin. Published by Cambridge University Press. © Cambridge University Press 2008.

Table 9.1   Indications for esophageal stent placement

- Malignant esophageal obstruction [5,26,28,29,30,31]
- Tracheoesophageal fistulae [32,33]
- Primary or secondary tumors within the mediastinum causing extrinsic esophageal compression [34]
- Esophageal perforation [26,28,35,36]
- Treatment of symptomatic malignant gastroesophageal anastomotic leaks [37]
- Anastomotic tumor recurrence following surgery [6]

Indications for placement

These are listed in Table 9.1.

Contraindications

There are no *absolute* contraindications for esophageal stent placement, but there are several relative contraindications that include

- INR > 1.5 and platelets
- recent high dose of chemo/radiotherapy (3–6 weeks) because of increased risk of hemorrhage and perforation [38,39];
- severely ill patients with limited life expectancy;
- obstructive lesion of the stomach and/or of the small bowel due to peritoneal seeding;
- severe tracheal compression that would be made worse by esophageal intubation; and
- very high stenoses, close to the vocal cords.

Current stents and stent selection

Three main groups of self-expanding stents are available, which differ in material, shape, and radial force. These are Nitinol stents (Figure 9.1) [23,24], stainless steel stents, and plastic stents.

There are several types of devices available such as the esophageal Wallstent (Boston Scientific, Natick, Massachusetts) [7,40,41,42], the Ultraflex stent (Boston

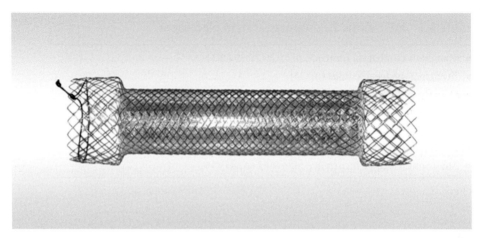

Figure 9.1 A retrievable Nitinol esophageal stent, Niti-S (Taewoong Medical, Seoul).

Scientific) [7,28,43,44], the Gianturco-Rösch Z stent with or without antireflux distal valve (William Cook Europe, Bjaeverskov, Denmark) [29,45,46,47], the EsophaCoil (IntraTherapeutics, St. Paul, Minnesota) [48,49], the Flamingo stent (Boston Scientific) [48], the FerX-Ella stent with antireflux distal valve (Radiologic Ltd.) [50], the Choo stent (Diagmed, UK) [51], the Memotherm (C.R. Bard, Germany) [42], the Song stent (Sooho Medi-tech, Korea) [52,53], and the Polyflex esophageal stent (Rusch®, Germany) [54,55,56].

All available types of stents can provide adequate relief of dysphagia caused by intrinsic esophageal tumors. The main factors influencing the choice of a stent are the location and the characteristics of the stricture.

Early covered stent designs were associated with high rates of migration, making it necessary to use uncovered devices when treating lesions at the cardia, in order to minimize the occurrence of this complication [26,28]. Current designs of covered stents incorporate features such as proximal flaring, partly uncovered portions, and placing the covering material on the inside, which reduce the rate of migration. Therefore, covered stents are usually preferred, as they minimize the risk of tumor ingrowth [57,58,59]. Covered esophageal stents should also be used in the palliation of tracheoesophageal and bronchoesophageal fistulae and leaks secondary to esophageal perforation [60,61]. Uncovered stents are useful in patients with extrinsic compression, a markedly dilated esophagus or with gastric pull-up. When the esophagus is very dilated, the use of an uncovered stent allows liquid or semisolid food to pass through the mesh of the device as it projects into the esophageal lumen and also reduces the risk of migration.

In the upper esophagus, the soft, covered Ultraflex stent or retrievable devices, which have greater flexibility and a weaker radial force, are preferred, as they are less likely than stiffer devices to cause pain and are easier to reposition.

Stenting across the gastroesophageal junction can result in severe gastroesophageal reflux. Frequently, such patients are prophylactically prescribed a proton pump inhibitor such as omeprazole (Losec). An alternative approach involves the use of a valved stent [50,59], which is designed to prevent reflux. In patients with significant dysphagia caused by potentially resectable esophageal cancer who need to gain weight prior to surgery whilst the tumor is being downstaged with chemotherapy, the placement of retrievable SEMS can be very helpful.

Technique of stent insertion

Esophageal stents can be inserted under fluoroscopic guidance alone, although many endoscopists prefer to combine endoscopic and fluoroscopic methods. The radiological technique has been well documented [5,6]. After an esophagogram has been obtained to delineate the site and length of the stricture (Figure 9.2a), the patient is placed in the left lateral position on a fluoroscopy table. The pharynx is anesthetized with lidocaine spray, and a catheter is passed perorally into the esophagus. The stricture is crossed with standard catheter guide-wire techniques. The stricture may be predilated to 14 mm, which facilitates introduction of the delivery system, allows rapid expansion of the stent, and enables more accurate placement (Figure 9.2b). A stent of appropriate size and length is advanced across the stricture on its delivery system and is usually deployed in such a way that slightly more of the stent is above the stricture than below it, to reduce the risk of distal migration. After stent deployment, contrast medium is injected via a catheter to confirm patency of the stent and exclude the presence of perforation [5,23]. However, this initial catheter study may miss a perforation in the nondependent wall of the esophagus. Therefore, a second esophagogram should be carried out when the patient has recovered from the sedation to exclude a small perforation and to confirm that the stent has maintained its position (Figure 9.2c).

Success rates

The technical success rate of stent placement under fluoroscopy guidance approximates 100%. The improvement in swallowing is best indicated by means of the dysphagia score, which has five grades: grade 0, normal diet; grade 1, some solid

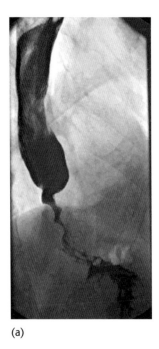

(a)

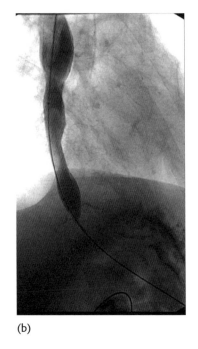

(b)

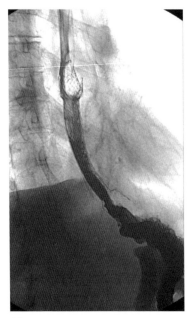

(c)

Figure 9.2 Patient with adenocarcinoma requiring palliative stent insertion: (a) contrast swallow demonstrating a typical tight esophageal malignant stricture; (b) 14 mm dilated balloon deployed across stricture for predilatation; and (c) swallow showing good flow of contrast through esophagus after stent insertion.

food; grade 2, semisolids only; grade 3, liquids only; grade 4, complete dysphagia. In most patients, the dysphagia score decreases by at least one grade [5,6,26,28,29,30,31]. Although most patients die during the following 4 months, their quality of life improves substantially [23].

In the palliation of malignant esophagorespiratory fistulae and perforations, covered metallic stents have a clinical success rate of 95–100% [60,61].

Complications

The main procedural complications are perforation, aspiration, hemorrhage, and stent misplacement.

Postprocedural complications include perforation, hemorrhage, stent migration, pain/sensation of a foreign body, tumor ingrowth/overgrowth, stent occlusion due to a bolus of food, reflux, esophagitis, fistulation, and sepsis.

Procedure-related complications are lower in patients treated with metallic stents than in those treated with the rigid plastic endoprostheses. Hemorrhage has been reported in 3–8% but is usually mild and self-limiting [26,28,29,30,31,35]. In those rare cases of severe hemorrhage, angiography with embolization of the bleeding vessel with Gelfoam or coils can be undertaken. Fistulae and perforation attributable to stent insertion are uncommon [36]. Early chest pain occurs in most patients, but prolonged pain occurs in fewer than 13% of patients [28]. Pain is more severe in patients with high strictures and when using large-diameter stents [31]. The incidence of migration when using uncovered stents is less than 3% when the stent is within the esophagus and increasing to 6% for stents placed across the cardia [7,26]. The migration rate of early designs of covered stents, especially when positioned across the cardia, was 25–32% [26,28,59], but with newer devices this complication is observed in fewer than 5% of patients. Partially migrated stents can be stabilized in position by coaxially inserting another stent, which overlaps the upper half of the migrated stent. If there is complete migration of the stent, the lesion is treated by insertion of a new stent. Stents migrating into the stomach can be left in place in asymptomatic patients. However, if the patient has pain, the stent can be removed via a gastrostomy, surgical incision, or endoscopically [62]. Tumor ingrowth occurs in 17–36% [28,30] of uncovered stents but is rarely seen with covered stents [7,26,43]. Recurrent dysphagia as a result of tumor overgrowth has been reported in up to 60% of the patients followed up for long enough [63]. Tumor ingrowth or overgrowth can be treated by coaxial stenting.

Metallic stent insertion has a very low procedural mortality rate, between 0 and 1.4% [26,28,29,30,31,35]. Stent insertion in patients who have had recent radiotherapy or in whom radiotherapy is given immediately after the insertion of a stent is associated with an increased rate of complications, particularly hemorrhage [38,39,64,65,66,67]. We recommend an interval of at least 4–6 weeks after radiotherapy and stent insertion.

Conclusions

The available esophageal stents provide palliation in esophageal cancer, but the most urgent need is for a temporary device that can be used in patients who are being downstaged prior to surgery [68] without the need to use a removable stent, which entails an additional procedure for the patient. Biodegradable devices would meet this need, and some work is being undertaken to develop such stents.

REFERENCES

1. P. C. Enzinger and R. J. Mayer. Medical progress: Esophageal cancer. *N Engl J Med*, **349**:23 (2003), 2241–52.
2. P. Pisani, D. M. Parkin, F. Bray, *et al.* Estimates of the worldwide mortality from 25 cancers in 1990. *Int J Cancer*, **83** (1999), 18–29.
3. A. K. Kubba and N. Krasner. An update in the palliative management of malignant dysphagia. *Eur J Surg Oncol*, **26** (2000), 116–29.
4. R. Mason. Palliation of oesophageal cancer. *Surg Oncol*, **10** (2001), 123–6.
5. R. Morgan and A. Adam. Esophageal stents – An update. *Semin Intervent Radiol*, **18**:3 (2001), 251–64.
6. S. H. Lee. The role of oesophageal stenting in the non-surgical management of oesophageal strictures. *Br J Radiol*, **74** (2001), 891–900.
7. A. Adam, J. Ellul, A. F. Watkinson, *et al.* Palliation of inoperable esophageal carcinoma: a prospective randomised trial of laser therapy and stent placement. *Radiology*, **202** (1997), 344–8.
8. A. M. Gevers, E. Macken, M. Hiele, *et al.* A comparison of laser therapy, plastic stents and expandable metal stents for palliation of malignant dysphagia in patients without a fistula. *Gastrointest Endosc*, **48** (1998), 383–8.
9. D. S. Tan, R. C. Mason, A. Adam, *et al.* Minimally invasive therapy for advanced oesophageal malignancy. *Clin Radiol*, **51** (1996), 828–36.

10. S. K. Heier, K. A. Rothman, L. M. Heier, *et al.* Photodynamic therapy for obstructing oesophageal cancer: light dosimetry and randomised comparisons with Nd:YAG laser therapy. *Gastroenterology*, **109** (1995), 63–72.

11. C. J. Lightdale, S. K. Heier, and M. E. Manon. Photodynamic therapy with porfimer sodium versus thermal ablation with Nd:YAG laser for palliation of esophageal cancer: a multi-centre randomised trial. *Gastrointest Endosc*, **42** (1995), 507–12.

12. J. D. Luketich, N. A. Christine, P. O. Buenaventura, *et al.* Endoscopic photodynamic therapy for obstructing oesophageal cancer: 77 cases over a 2 year period. *Surg Endosc*, **14** (2000), 653–7.

13. R. Earlam and J. R. Cunha-Melo. Oesophageal squamous cell carcinoma. A critical review of radiotherapy. *Br J Surg*, **67** (1980), 457–61.

14. A. Bamias, M. Hill, D. Cunningham, *et al.* Epirubicin, cisplatin and protracted venous infusional 5 fluorouracil for oesophagogastric adenocarcinoma: response, toxicity, quality of life and survival. *Cancer*, **77** (1996), 1978–85.

15. M. Highley, F. Parnis, G. A. Trotter, *et al.* Combination chemotherapy with epirubicin, cisplatin and 5 fluorouracil for the palliation of advanced gastric and oesophageal adenocarcinoma. *Br J Surg*, **81** (1994), 1763–5.

16. L. U. Nwokolo, J. J. Payne-James, D. B. A. Silk, *et al.* Palliation of malignant dysphagia by ethanol induced tumour necrosis. *Gut*, **35** (1994), 299–303.

17. J. J. Payne-James, R. C. Spiller, and J. J. Misiewicz. Use of ethanol induced tumour necrosis to palliate dysphagia in patients with esophagogastric cancer. *Gastrointest Endosc*, **36** (1990), 43–6.

18. S. C. S. Chung, H. T. Leong, and C. Y. C. Choi. Palliation of malignant esophageal obstruction by endoscopic alcohol injection. *Endoscopy*, **26** (1994), 275–7.

19. H. Heindorff, M. Wojdemann, T. Bisgaard, *et al.* Endoscopic palliation of inoperable cancer of the esophagus or cardia by organ electrocoagulation. *Scand J Gastroenterol*, **33** (1998), 21–3.

20. T. M. Mekhail, D. J. Adelstein, L. A. Rybicki, *et al.* Enteral nutrition during the treatment of head and neck carcinoma: is a percutaneous endoscopic gastrostomy tube preferable to nasogastric tube? *Cancer*, **91**:9 (2001), 1785–90.

21. N. Magne, P. Y. Marcy, C. Foa, *et al.* Comparison between nasogastric tube feeding and percutaneous fluoroscopic gastrostomy in advanced head and neck cancer patients. *Eur Arch Otorhinolaryngol*, **258**:2 (2001), 89–92.

22. C. Ripamonti, B. T. Gemlo, F. Bozzetti, *et al.* Role of enteral nutrition in advanced cancer patients: indications and contraindications of the different techniques employed. *Tumori*, **82** (1996), 302–8.

23. C. A. O'Donell, G. M. Fullarton, E. Watt, *et al.* Randomized clinical trial comparing self-expanding metallic stents with plastic endoprostheses in the palliation of oesophageal cancer. *Br J Surg*, **89** (2002), 985–92.

24. F. Mosca, A. Consoli, A. Stracqualursi, *et al.* Comparative retrospective study on the use of plastic prostheses and self-expanding metal stents in the palliative treatment of malignant strictures of the esophagus and cardia. *Dis Esophagus*, **16** (2003), 119–25.

25. G. D. De Palma, E. di Matteo, E. Romano, *et al.* Plastic prosthesis versus expandable metal stents for palliation of inoperable oesophageal thoracic carcinoma: a controlled prospective study. *Gastrointest Endosc*, **43** (1996), 478–82.

26. W. Cwikiel, K. G. Tranberg, M. Cwikiel, *et al.* Malignant dysphagia: palliation with oesophageal stents – long term results in 100 patients. *Radiology*, **207** (1998), 513–18.

27. C. J. Symonds. A case of malignant stricture of the oesophagus illustrating the use of a new form of oesophageal catheter. *Trans Clin Soc Lond*, **18** (1885), 155–8.

28. B. Acunas, I. Rozanes, S. Akpinar, *et al.* Palliation of malignant esophageal strictures with self-expanding Nitinol stents: drawbacks and complications. *Radiology*, **199** (1996), 648–52.

29. H. U. Laasch, D. A. Nicholson, C. L. Kay, *et al.* The clinical effectiveness of the Gianturco oesophageal stent in malignant oesophageal obstruction. *Clin Radiol*, **53** (1998), 666–72.

30. G. Costamagna, M. Marchese, and F. Iacopin. Self-expanding stents in oesophageal cancer. *Eur J Gastroenterol Hepatol*, **18** (2006), 1177–80.

31. H. Y. Song, Y. S. Do, Y. M. Han, *et al.* Covered, expandable oesophageal metallic stent tubes: experience in 119 patients. *Radiology*, **207** (1998), 513–18.

32. A. F. Watkinson, J. Ellul, K. Entwistle, *et al.* Plastic-covered metallic endoprostheses in the management of esophageal perforation in patients with esophageal carcinoma. *Clin Radiol*, **50** (1995), 304–9.

33. Y. S. Do, H. Y. Song, B. H. Lee, *et al.* Esophagorespiratory fistula associated with esophageal cancer: treatment with a Gianturco stent tube. *Radiology*, **187** (1993), 673–7.

34. N. K. Gupta, C. E. Boylan, R. Razzaq, *et al.* Self expanding oesophageal metal stents for the palliation of dysphagia due to extrinsic compression. *Eur Radiol*, **9** (1999), 1893–7.

35. R. R. Saxon, R. E. Barton, and J. Rösch. Complications of oesophageal stenting and balloon dilatation. *Semin Intervent Radiol*, **11** (1994), 276–82.

36. M. Faruggia, R. A. Morgan, J. A. Latham, *et al.* Perforation of the esophagus secondary to insertion of covered Wallstent endoprostheses. *Cardiovasc Intervent Radiol*, **20** (1994), 428–30.

37. M. Tyrell, G. Trotter, A. Adam, *et al.* Incidence and management of laser-associated oesophageal perforation. *Br J Surg*, **82** (1995), 1257–8.

38. Y. Nishimura, K. Nagata, S. Katano, *et al.* Severe complications in advanced esophageal cancer treated with radiotherapy after intubation of esophageal stents: a questionnaire survey of the Japanese Society for Esophageal Diseases. *Int J Radiat Oncol Biol Phys*, **56**:5 (2003), 1327–32.

39. M. Yakami, M. Mitsumori, H. Sai, *et al.* Development of severe complications caused by stent placement followed by definitive radiation therapy for T4 esophageal cancer. *Int J Clin Oncol*, **8**:6 (2003), 395–8.

40. A. F. Watkinson, J. Ellul, K. Entwisle, *et al.* Oesophageal carcinoma: initial results of palliative treatment with covered self-expanding endoprostheses. *Radiology*, **195** (1995), 821–7.

41. A. Schamassmann, C. Meyenberger, J. Knuchel, *et al.* Self-expanding metal stents in malignant esophageal obstruction: a comparison between two stent types. *Am J Gastroenterol*, **92** (1997), 400–6.

42. I. Raijman, I. Siddiqui, J. Ajani, *et al.* Palliation of malignant dysphagia and fistulae with coated expandable metal stents: experience with 101 patients. *Gastrointest Endosc*, **48** (1998), 172–9.

43. F. W. Winkelbauer, R. Schofl, B. Niederle, *et al.* Palliative treatment of obstructing esophageal cancer with nitinol stents: value, safety, and long-term results. *AJR Am J Roentgenol*, **166** (1996), 79–84.

44. G. J. O'Sullivan and A. Grundy. Palliation of malignant dysphagia with expanding metal stents. *J Vasc Intervent Radiol*, **10** (1999), 346–51.

45. C. D. Roseveare, P. Patel, N. Simmonds, *et al.* Metal stents improve dysphagia, nutrition and survival in malignant oesophageal stenosis: a ramdomised controlled trial comparing modified Gianturco Z stents with plastic Atkinson tubes. *Eur J Gastroenterol Hepatol*, **10** (1998), 653–7.

46. P. D. Siersema, C. J. Hop, J. Dees, *et al.* Coated self expanding stent versus latex prostheses for esophagogastric cancer with special reference to prior radiation and chemotherapy: a controlled prospective study. *Gastrointest Endosc*, **46** (1998), 113–19.

47. R. Kozarek, S. Raltz, W. R. Brugge, *et al.* Prospective multicentre trial of oesophageal Z-stent placement for malignant dysphagia and trancheoesophageal fistula. *Gastrointest Endosc*, **44**(1996), 562–7.

48. D. Wengrower, A. Fiorini, J. Valero, *et al.* EsophaCoil: long term results in 81 patients. *Gastrointest Endosc*, **48** (1998), 376–82.

49. E. Olsen, R. Thyregaard, J. Kill, *et al.* Esophageal expanding stent in the management of patients with non-resectable malignant esophageal or cardiac neoplasm: a prospective study. *Endoscopy*, **31** (1999), 417–20.

50. K. S. Dua, R. Kozarek, J. Kim, *et al.* Self expanding metal esophageal stent with anti-reflux mechanism. *Gastrointest Endosc*, **53** (2001), 603–13.

51. H. Y. Song, H. Y. Jung, S. I. Park, *et al.* Covered retrievable expandable Nitinol stents in patients with benign esophageal strictures: initial experience. *Radiology*, **217** (2000), 551–7.

52. J. F. Bartelsman, M. J. Bruno, A. J. Jensema, *et al.* Palliation of patients with esophagogastric neoplasm by insertion of a covered expandable modified Gianturco-Z endoprosthesis: experiences in 153 patients. *Gastrointest Endosc*, **51** (2000), 134–8.

53. H. Y. Song, S. I. Park, H. Y. Jung, *et al.* Benign and malignant esophageal strictures: treatment with a polyurethane-covered retrievable expandable metallic stent. *Radiology*, **203** (1997), 747–52.

54. J. Broto, M. Asensio, and J. M. Vernet. Results of a new technique in the treatment of severe esophageal stenosis in children: polyflex stents. *J Pediatr Gastroenterol Nutr*, **37** (2003), 203–6.

55. G. Costamagna, S. K. Shak, A. Tringali, *et al.* Prospective evaluation of a new self-expanding plastic stent for inoperable esophageal strictures. *Surg Endosc*, **17** (2003), 891–5.

56. A. J. Dormann, P. Eisandrath, B. Wigginghaus, *et al.* Palliation of esophageal carcinoma with a new self-expanding plastic stent. *Endoscopy*, **35** (2003), 207–11.

57. A. Adam, R. Morgan, J. Ellul, *et al.* A new design of the esophageal Wallstent endoprosthesis resistant to distal migration. *AJR Am J Roentgenol*, **170** (1998), 1477–82.

58. T. Sabharwal, M. S. Hamady, S. Chui, *et al.* A randomized prospective comparison of the Flamingo Wallstent and Ultraflex stent for palliation of dysphagia associated with lower third oesophageal carcinoma. *Gut*, **52** (2003), 922–6.

59. M. Kocher, M. Dlouhy, C. Neoral, *et al.* Esophageal stent with antireflux valve for tumors involving the cardia: work in progress. *J Vasc Intervent Radiol*, **9** (1998), 1007–10.

60. A. A. Nicholson, C. M. S. Royston, K. Wedgewood, *et al.* Palliation of malignant oesophageal perforation and proximal oesophageal malignant dysphagia with covered metal stents. *Clin Radiol*, **50** (1995), 11–14.

61. R. A. Morgan, J. P. M. Ellul, E. R. E. Denton, *et al.* Malignant esophageal fistulas and perforations: management with plastic-covered metallic endoprostheses. *Radiology*, **204** (1997), 527–32.

62. T. Sabharwal, J. P. Morales, R. Salter, *et al.* Esophageal cancer: self-expanding metallic stents. *Abdom Imaging*, **29** (2004), 1–9.

63. W. Mayoral, D. Fleischer, J. Salcedo, *et al.* Non-malignant obstruction is a common problem with metal stents in the treatment of oesophageal cancer. *Gastrointest Endosc*, **51** (2000), 556–9.

64. P. D. Siersema, W. C. Hop, J. Dees, H. W. Tilanus, and M. van Blankenstein. Coated self-expanding metal stents versus latex prostheses for esophagogastric cancer with special reference to prior radiation and chemotherapy: a controlled, prospective study. *Gastrointest Endosc*, **47** (1998), 113–20.

65. P. D. Siersema, W. C. Hop, M. van Blankenstein, *et al.* A comparison of 3 types of covered metal stents for the palliation of patients with dysphagia caused by 25 esophagogastric carcinoma: a prospective, randomized study. *Gastrointest Endosc*, **54** (2001), 145–53.

66. M. Y. Homs, B. E. Hansen, M. van Blankenstein, *et al.* Prior radiation and/or chemotherapy has no effect on the outcome of metal stent placement for oesophagogastric carcinoma. *Eur J Gastroenterol Hepatol*, **16** (2004), 163–70.

67. J. H. Shin, H. Y. Song, J. H. Kim, *et al.* Comparison of temporary and permanent stent placement with concurrent radiation therapy in patients with esophageal carcinoma. *J Vasc Intervent Radiol*, **16** (2005), 67–74.

68. T. Sabharwal, J. P. Morales, F. G. Irani, and A. Adam. Quality improvement guidelines for placement of esophageal stents. *Cardiovasc Intervent Radiol*, **28** (2005), 284–8.

Lasers in Esophageal Cancer

Laurence B. Lovat

Introduction

Lasers are sophisticated sources of monochromatic light. In the near-infrared part of the optical spectrum, laser light penetrates living tissue well and can be transmitted via thin, flexible fibers through the working channel of endoscopes. High-power shots of light turn into heat, which vaporizes tissue and coagulates the underlying layers. This effectively debulks advanced cancers. At much lower powers, it is possible to coagulate a larger volume of tissue without vaporization.

Laser can also deliver a *photodynamic* effect where there is no increase in tissue temperature, but the light activates a previously administered photosensitizing drug. This causes the release of highly reactive singlet oxygen, which causes cell death by necrosis and apoptosis over a prolonged period. This can be used to completely eradicate small tumors (Table 10.1).

Palliation of advanced cancers

Most patients with cancer of the esophagus or gastric cardia present with locally advanced disease and therefore are unsuitable for surgery. One of the main aims of treatment is to relieve dysphagia as simply and rapidly as possible [1]. The most widely used endoscopic approach is tumor dilatation and insertion of an expanding metal stent although many oncologists do not advocate endoscopic therapy at all, relying on radiotherapy or chemotherapy to improve dysphagia. It is clear that oncological therapy alone is more suitable only for mild dysphagia, but for patients who are only able to tolerate liquids, an endoscopic therapy is better [2]. Stents are, however, far from ideal, with only 70% of patients being able to eat reasonably

Carcinoma of the Esophagus, ed. Sheila C. Rankin. Published by Cambridge University Press. © Cambridge University Press 2008.

Table 10.1 Laser effects used in gastroenterology

Laser effect	Clinical use
High-power thermal	Hemostasis
	Cutting or debulking of tissue by vaporization and coagulation
Low-power thermal (interstitial laser photocoagulation [ILP])	Gentle coagulation of lesions within solid organs
Photochemical (photodynamic therapy [PDT])	Nonthermal destruction of tissue by activation of a previously administered photosensitizing drug
Pulsed shock wave	Fragmentation of gall stones

normally. Up to 40% require further intervention, and intractable pain occurs in 10% of patients after stent insertion [3,4].

Laser therapy has been shown to improve dysphagia to a similar degree as stents, and it does not cause pain. During endoscopy, high-power, thermal lasers can be used to vaporize nodules of exophytic tumor under direct vision. Underlying tumor is also coagulated. This relieves obstruction and reduces blood loss (Figure 10.1). The incidence of complications is low, although it often takes several treatments to achieve optimum recanalization. There is minimal risk to operators with video scopes, although filters are required to protect the chips in the camera.

Complications are rare [5], but the disadvantage is that laser therapy alone has to be repeated on average every 5 weeks. The addition of a palliative dose of external beam radiotherapy can increase this to 9 weeks [6], and a single fraction of brachytherapy (intraluminal radiotherapy) will bring relief of dysphagia for a median of 5 months [7]. Recent data have also shown that brachytherapy as a monotherapy brings more long-term benefits than stenting [8], although initial relief of dysphagia is slow. Our own experience suggests that initial laser followed by brachytherapy gives both immediate relief from dysphagia and long-term benefits [7].

The relative merits of lasers and stents are summarized in Table 10.2. Common sense dictates that the two approaches are complementary rather than competitive. An eccentric, exophytic tumor is best debulked with the laser, whereas a circumferential tumor with little exophytic component is best stented. A fistula must be stented, whereas high cervical tumors can seldom be stented. What little data there are on comparative costs suggest that the lifetime treatment costs are similar for each of these approaches [9].

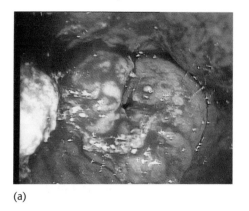

(a)

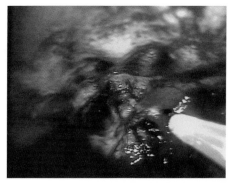

(b)

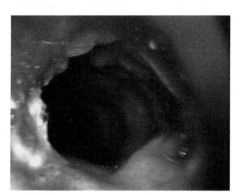

(c)

Figure 10.1 Advanced, obstructing carcinoma of the esophagus: (a) at presentation; (b) during laser therapy; and (c) after two endoscopic laser treatments. The esophageal lumen has been reopened and the patient's dysphagia has been relieved.

A future direction may be the combination of laser palliation of dysphagia with radical chemoradiotherapy for inoperable patients. Many patients with advanced disease present with severe malnutrition caused by their dysphagia. Radical treatment is not possible in a cachectic patient, but if dysphagia is overcome, patients regain weight and are able to tolerate intensive therapy. Long-term data are lacking, but early results suggest that this approach can lead to prolonged survival in at least some patients who have previously been thought to be terminally ill [10].

Photodynamic therapy

Photodynamic therapy (PDT) is an attractive option for treating small tumors of the gastrointestinal tract in patients who are unsuitable for surgery. Whilst causing localized tissue necrosis, it does not affect collagen, so the risk of perforation of the

Table 10.2   Comparison of modalities for palliation of malignant dysphagia

	Laser	Self-expanding metal stent
Technique	Basically safe (risk of perforation if dilatation also needed)	Usually safe and easy to insert
Cost	High setup cost Low patient costs	High cost
Contraindications	Fistula No endoscopic target	High lesion Tracheal compression Care with lesions crossing cardia
Dysphagia after therapy	Variable, can be close to normal	Variable, can be close to normal
Repeat therapy	Possible. Usually required after 4–6 weeks	Difficult to adjust once inserted. Second stent or laser debulking for tumor overgrowth
Enhancement of dysphagia relief with radiotherapy	Yes	No

wall of the gastrointestinal tract is very low [11,12]. In 123 patients with early esophageal cancers treated with PDT using the photosensitizer porfimer sodium (Photofrin), a complete local response was seen in 87% at 6 months [13]. The disease-specific survival at 5 years was 75%. We have similar experience using the newer drug Foscan [14]. PDT can be applied at any endoscopically accessible site, but it cannot treat any lesion that has spread beyond the site of origin as, for example, to local lymph nodes. PDT has side effects including esophageal stricturing as well as photosensitivity that may be prolonged; however, newer drugs may overcome this problem.

PDT has been proposed for the palliation of advanced malignant dysphagia. Although it does provide some relief in this situation, there are very few cases that can be helped by PDT if thermal laser therapy or stent insertion fail, and it is certainly not desirable to make patients photosensitive for much of their remaining life [5,15]. In general terms, it seems more logical to limit the use of PDT to early esophageal cancers.

Conclusions

Thermal laser is an established tool for endoscopic palliation of advanced gastro-intestinal tract cancers. It has a complementary role to stents and is likely to bring benefit to patients as part of multimodality treatment together with radiotherapy. PDT is an alternative laser therapy but probably has limited use in palliating advanced cancer.

REFERENCES

1. L. B. Lovat and S. G. Bown. Lasers in gastroenterology. *World J Gastroenterol*, **15** (2001), 317–23.

2. R. J. L. Caspers, K. Welvaart, R. J. Verkes, J. Hermans, and J. W. H. Leer. The effect of radio-therapy on dysphagia and survival in patients with esophageal cancer. *Radiother Oncol*, **12** (1988), 15–23.

3. W. Cwikiel, K. G. Tranberg, M. Cwikiel, and R. Lillo-Gil. Malignant dysphagia: palliation with esophageal stents – long-term results in 100 patients. *Radiology*, **207** (1998), 513–18.

4. L. B. Lovat, N. Mathou, S. M. Thorpe, *et al.* Relief of dysphagia with self expanding metal stents is far from perfect. *Gut*, **46** (2000), W22.

5. W. H. Allum, S. M. Griffin, A. Watson, *et al.* Guidelines for the management of oesophageal and gastric cancer. *Gut*, **50**:Suppl. 5 (2002), v1–23.

6. I. R. Sargeant, J. S. Tobias, G. Blackman, *et al.* Radiotherapy enhances laser palliation of malig-nant dysphagia: A randomised study. *Gut*, **40** (1997), 362–9.

7. G. M. Spencer, S. M. Thorpe, G. M. Blackman, *et al.* Laser augmented by brachytherapy versus laser alone in the palliation of adenocarcinoma of the oesophagus and cardia: a randomised study. *Gut*, **50** (2002), 224–7.

8. M. Y. Homs, E. W. Steyerberg, W. M. Eijkenboom, *et al.* Single-dose brachytherapy versus metal stent placement for the palliation of dysphagia from oesophageal cancer: multicentre rando-mised trial. *Lancet*, **364** (2004), 1497–504.

9. M. J. Sculpher, I. R. Sargeant, L. A. Loizou, *et al.* A cost analysis of Nd:YAG laser ablation versus endoscopic intubation for the palliation of malignant dysphagia. *Eur J Cancer*, **31** (1995), 1640–6.

10. L. B. Lovat, C. H. Bridgewater, T. Evans, *et al.* A new approach to the treatment of inoperable carcinoma of the oesophagus: Laser and radical chemoradiation therapy. *Gut*, **48**:Suppl. 1 (2001), A9.

11. T. J. Dougherty, C. J. Gomer, B. W. Henderson, *et al.* Photodynamic therapy. *J Natl Cancer Inst*, **90** (1998), 889–905.

12. H. Barr, C. J. Tralau, P. B. Boulos, *et al.* The contrasting mechanisms of colonic collagen damage between photodynamic therapy and thermal injury. *Photochem Photobiol*, **46** (1987), 795–800.

13. A. Sibille, C. Descamps, P. Jonard, *et al.* Endoscopic Nd:YAG treatment of superficial gastric carcinoma: experience in 18 Western inoperable patients. *Gastrointest Endosc*, **42** (1995), 340–5.

14. L. B. Lovat, N. F. Jamieson, M. R. Novelli, *et al.* Photodynamic therapy with m-tetrahydroxyphenyl chlorin for high-grade dysplasia and early cancer in Barrett's columnar lined esophagus. *Gastrointest Endosc*, **62** (2005), 617–23.

15. S. G. Bown and C. E. Millson. Photodynamic therapy in gastroenterology. *Gut*, **41** (1997), 5–7.

Index

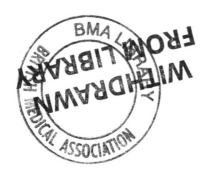